Raising Healthy Pets

Insights of a Holistic Veterinarian

Norman Ralston, D.V.M.
with Gale Jack

One Peaceful World Press
Becket, Massachusetts

Raising Healthy Pets
© 1996 by Norman Ralston and Gale Jack

For further information on mail-order sales, wholesale or retail dis-
counts, distribution, translations, and foreign rights, please contact
the publisher:

One Peaceful World Press
P. O. Box 10
Leland Road
Becket, MA 01223
U.S.A.

Telephone (413) 623-2322
Fax (413) 623-8827

First Edition: September 1996
10 9 8 7 6 5 4 3 2 1

ISBN 1–882984–22–6
Printed in U.S.A.

Contents

1. Getting into Macrobiotics   5

2. Growing Up in East Texas   14

3. Learning from My Grandmother   22

4. From the Family Farm to the Factory Farm   30

5. The Human-Animal Bond   38

6. How to Keep Dogs and Cats Healthy   50

7. Prenatal Care and Birthing   60

8. Kitten and Puppy Care   70

9. Determining What the Adult Animal Should Eat   84

10. Grooming, Exercising, Bathing, Immunizing, Neutering,
    and Spaying   99

Resources   110
Recommended Reading   111
About the Authors   112

Acknowledgements

The authors would like to express their deep gratitude to Ann Fawcett, who originally conceived this project. Ann taped and transcribed the hundreds of hours of interviews with Dr. Ralston on which *Raising Healthy Pets* is based. They are also grateful to Alex Jack and Janet Barton for help with reviewing and editing the manuscript.

The companion book in this series, *Healing Your Pet Naturally* by Dr. Ralston, focuses on treating common conditions and chronic diseases in dogs and cats, and will be published by One Peaceful World Press in the near future.

1
Getting into Macrobiotics

My path to becoming a holistic veterinarian started with an interest in alternative healing methods. In the early 1970s, I attended a conference of the American Animal Hospital Association in San Francisco and learned that a couple of young men were doing something that I had tried unsuccessfully to do for years. They had used acupuncture to improve a horse's breathing and played a tape recording that showed the change. I was impressed. Back home, I felt I would like to know more about Oriental medicine.

I called Stephen Uprichard of the East West Foundation. He said they had a course in acupuncture that lasted for several months and would be happy to have me come. But it would have been difficult to get away from work for that length of time, so I asked if they ever came across the country to teach. He said that a weekend seminar could be arranged for about a thousand dollars. I thought, "This will be no problem. I'll get together a bunch of other veterinarians, and we can all share the expense." But I ran up against a stone wall. I didn't even get one vet. Then I opened it up to the public. One young woman who brings her dog into my veterinary clinic joined in. She was an airline stewardess and on maternity leave at the time.

Four or five months later, Stephen Uprichard came down to Dallas, and by that time others had signed up for the course. He taught primarily acupressure massage rather than acupuncture, but we learned the philosophy behind Oriental medicine. He divided us into pairs and had us find the points common to acupressure, acupuncture, and other Far Eastern therapies. While he was here, I tried to gather as much information as I could, and what I learned spurred my further interest.

Shortly after that, I heard of a new group of veterinarians interested in Oriental healing. Out of these meetings the International Veterinary Acupuncture Society (IVAS) developed. We hired people to teach us. Some came from as far away as China. At one time, we had people from both the People's Republic and Taiwan instructing us. Dr. Wong, a Chinese-American acupuncturist from Denver, was in charge of the arrangements. Because of the political hostility between the two Chinas at that time, he sat the people from the People's Republic and from Taiwan with their backs to each other so they wouldn't have to communicate.

Our meetings were held in rented facilities at Purdue University in Indiana. They had a school of veterinary medicine, and we offered to let their staff attend our courses for free. Our group was well organized. We would meet every month for four days, and after the lectures we would go over to the veterinary school and practice what we had learned on some of the animals. At one class, Dr. Kaufbauer, an instructor from Vienna, shaved a cow to demonstrate to us the acupuncture points. Out of the group, at least ten veterinarians became nationally and internationally known. People came from all over the world to study and exchange ideas. In my own case, this education led me to look into the role of diet and nutrition in the conditions of the animals I was treating. I began to realize that food was causing many of their problems—problems I had never seen in the farm animals I grew up working with. I began to change my own diet as well.

Like many all-American, red-blooded Texans, I was a big steak-and-potatoes person for many years. I worked hard and felt that rich food was one of the compensations that life owed me. I bought premium cuts of beef and ate at fancy restaurants. I even had a special butcher in Oak Cliff from whom

I got the best beef money could buy. I used to get these thick steaks and barbecue them Texas style over a pit in the backyard. Sometimes I cooked them in the oven. I fixed meat like this every day.

Meanwhile, I started attending a church in Dallas oriented toward natural living. It was called the Today Church, and many of the people who went there were eating raw foods, juices, and herbs. Someone gave me one of the first copies of the *East West Journal*. I read that and began to frequent health food stores and pick up books on alternative lifestyles and philosophies. For a while, I was heavily involved with the Edgar Cayce materials.

About that time, my first wife and I separated, and I had the children with me. I cooked for them and decided to prepare meat only two days a week to save time. The rest of the time I would have leftovers. But trying to keep things going—my work at the clinic, getting up and getting the children off to school, and cooking for everybody—proved to be too much of a chore. I noticed that I'd eat a big plate of meat and not feel well for the next twenty-four hours. When I was just eating leftovers—mostly vegetables—I felt better. I said to myself, "Hmm, I'll skip meat the second day, too." Soon I was eating meat just one day a week. I began to feel better and better. I wasn't so belligerent. I was able to get my work done more efficiently. It evolved naturally like that.

Then, on Oct. 7, 1977, I began to have a health crisis that led me to macrobiotics. I had just returned from an acupuncture seminar in Southern California. I got home and noticed a swelling on my side. Ever since I was a kid, there had been a little knot there, but it had never bothered me much. Then all of a sudden it began to grow and become more sensitive. I tried to ignore it, but by early December it had grown as big as a fist.

Toward the end of December, I tried to set up a consultation with Michio Kushi. I had previously attended a macrobiotic seminar sponsored by the East West Foundation in Amherst and knew that he was the best person to go to for advice. Unfortunately, he was very busy and a personal guidance session could not be set up for many months. I persisted, however, and flew to Boston hoping that he would see me. I approached Olivia Oredson, one of Michio's assistants. She called me one day at the hotel where I was staying and where Michio was scheduled to give a medical seminar. "Michio will stop and speak with you just a moment by the door," she said. I talked to him very briefly and showed him the growth on my side. He told me to observe the Standard Macrobiotic Diet and recommended some special condiments and side dishes. This began my introduction to umeboshi plums, daikon radish, and other exotic foods from the Far East that I had never heard of before. The names of these foods and the general philosophy of yin and yang were so foreign to me. I'd had a little exposure to macrobiotics at the seminar in Amherst, but then I was just investigating and didn't think it applied to me.

I turned completely serious. I went to some cooking classes and learned how to cook two or three main dishes, including pressure-cooked brown rice. I learned how to apply ginger compresses and taro potato plasters to the place on my side. The ginger compress went on first. The idea is to apply it as hot as you can stand in order to penetrate and get the blood and energy circulation going. After it became nice and red, I would apply the taro plaster. This is made by grating a hairy taro root, mixing it with a little flour and ginger, and making a poultice that is put over the swelling. The purpose of the taro plaster is to draw out stagnant and toxic material. But finding a taro root in Texas at the time was like finding teeth in a chicken's mouth. It was nearly impossible. So I took some taro home from Boston and eventually found a produce store that would order some for me from California. I kept at it and made sure they didn't run out.

About this time, my wife left for good. She had been up in Boston to help with my healing. She liked shiatsu massage and, in fact, became very good. She could even teach shiatsu. But macrobiotic cooking was a different matter. She considered herself the very best of cooks. Like a lot of other women who have been trained in the modern gourmet style of eating, this was an illusion, but she couldn't make the adjustment. One day I came home from the clinic and she had made me a dish with a lot of cheese. Dairy food is a "no-no" in the Standard Macrobiotic Diet, and I said, "I'm not eating that." This was the last straw in our relationship.

After she left, I continued cooking for myself. My menu was limited to the three dishes I had learned to prepare in Boston. I just rotated them, fixing one on one day, another the next. That's all I ate. I'm sure some of the people at the East West Foundation in Boston got tired of me calling and asking so many questions about my condition and when it would improve. The macrobiotic teachers kept telling me to be patient. Sometimes it took several months for a growth or tumor to discharge.

I continued to cook for myself as best I knew how. Keeping that thing on my side became difficult. It grew very painful for me just to shake hands with people. The vibration could drive you up the wall. I had to wear a big jacket to keep from hurting myself and no belt. After several weeks of this, I began noticing changes in the place on my side. It grew so sensitive that it took all the will power I could muster to apply the hot ginger compress. After about sixty days, I noticed a thin line developing on the growth. I called the EWF to ask if it would be all right to open it. They said it should naturally open and drain away, but the decision of whether to wait or hasten it along was up to me. I decided to wait. I just kept working with the diet and the home remedies.

Then one morning at the end of February I came in the house and noticed this terrible odor. I kept looking around for the source of the smell but couldn't find it. I had been wearing a large smock so that people wouldn't notice this orange-sized bulge sticking out of my side. When I began to take this smock off, I noticed that my side was draining and that it was the source of the odor. You can imagine the shock. Then I became terribly afraid that people would smell me. You can't imagine all the things I went through to try to keep the odor down. I even took to wearing a Kotex over the growth. I recognized the odor: it was like the odor of decaying human flesh, and I had smelled it in people with terminal cancer. It's an odor you never forget.

I continued working every day, but the smell could not

be concealed. Many well-meaning friends and associates tried to get me to seek medical attention. Earlier, before I had gone to Boston, I let one medical friend in Dallas look at it and he said, "Oh, man, we are going to take a biopsy." I said, "No, not yet." He said, "We'll find out what this thing is." I had always shied away from biopsies. In my experience, I'd seen that this procedure just sets the thing ablaze. It's like throwing gasoline on a fire.

Someone else asked me if I prayed. I replied, "Yes, I pray." They said, "How often?" I said, "Every breath." As far as I was concerned, every breath was a prayer. And they asked me if I said affirmations. I said, "Yes, I say affirmations." They said, "How often?" I said, "All the time. 'I'm young, whole, perfect, strong, powerful, loving, harmonious, and happy.'" I repeated that. I sang it. I whispered it. I shouted it. On the freeway when nobody could hear me, I screamed it.

Naturally I was heavily criticized by many people who couldn't understand why I didn't seek medical treatment. Somehow I managed to keep the odor under control and continued to function. Then one morning, I felt that my side was getting a little more loose. I put some pressure behind it with my thumb and the whole thing came out. It was the size of a green walnut.

I said, "Thank you, Father." There was a hole in my side that continued to drain for about ten days. The discharge relieved the discomfort. But the thing that was most impressive was that it seemed to lift the black cloud that hung around my shoulders. No matter how many affirmations or prayers I made, I had still been depressed. I had still felt angry and resentful. But these negative feelings all left when the growth came out. The whole world appeared brighter to me. The sky lightened up. Everything seemed to change for the better. That was around the beginning of March.

When macrobiotics worked so successfully on me, I decided to try it on animals. I started with food trials. Michio once said, "Food precedes thought." When I first heard that, I thought to myself, "That's a lie. I can think anything I want regardless of what I eat. And I can prove it doesn't work in my laboratory." In the clinic I had a client who had a poodle that was very aggressive. I believed it had been born with an aggressive personality and couldn't change. But to test Michio's theory, I talked the owner into feeding the dog what I called a very peaceful diet consisting mostly of whole grains and vegetables. I told the woman to bring the dog back in for a check-up in a month. Shortly after, she called and said, "You won't believe this durn dog." "Yeah?" I replied skeptically. "Yeah," she said, "he's changed a lot."

Now this was an animal with what I called a pathological thing about biting. He would bite people when there was no cause. You'd walk by him and he would snap and lunge. In other words, he wasn't a fear biter like a lot of dogs. This dog just seemed to enjoy biting on folks. If you were sitting on a couch in the house and that dog decided to get on the couch too, he would jump up and bite you so you would leave. He even bit family that way. At the clinic, we always had to restrain him when he came in.

But after the food trial, I could walk up and put my hands on this fierce little dog without so much as a nip. This was quite revealing. I began to think, "If I can do that, what other things can I do?" So I began to work with food and diet in my veterinary practice.

We haven't been one hundred percent successful. There's a time when things go beyond what natural healing is able to provide. But we have been able to use this dietary principle to help thousands and thousands of animals in the last ten or fifteen years. Not too long ago, for example, this Doberman pinscher was sent home to die. I could see that it had a tumor, and I estimated that with conventional medicine it might last four to six weeks. That was five and a half years ago—before macrobiotic treatment.

The owner recently brought the dog in. He was upset and crying, saying the cancer had returned. I said, "Wait a second. Let's take a look." I could find no evidence of a tumor. When I showed him, I said, "This dog is dying of old age." It was fifteen and a half; that's old for a Doberman pinscher. He finally reconciled himself to the fact that his dog's natural life span was over.

11

On the other hand, I have had cases where the tumor has come back. But most of the time when that happens, we find that the people are repeating past mistakes. One case in particular comes to mind. A lady came to see me. Her dog had a tumor on its side and was lethargic and didn't care what was going on. It was overweight and just blah. It reminded me of my former condition. The lady convinced me that she was very sincere about trying to save its life. She promised that she would do exactly what I told her.

I outlined a program of feeding the animal macrobiotically and showed her how to put on the taro plaster. She learned how to put a big body stocking on her dog. After several months, the dog began to get better. The tumor shrunk a little and became loose under the skin. I could feel that it was not attached to the body. I told her, "I think we could probably just make a slight incision in the skin and pull this thing out of here now, and put the taro right back on." She agreed, and we did that.

The dog changed from an animal not interested in anything to one that was interested in her toys again. If somebody came to visit, she would jump off the couch and bark at them in greeting. The animal's health and vitality returned, and she enjoyed a normal life for several years. Then once during a check-up, I examined her teeth and saw some old, ugly plaque from eating too much animal food. "Golly, she is still discharging this from the old diet," I thought. Then I said, "Wait a minute. She has been on this good diet for about three years now. She shouldn't be doing this."

I asked the lady very gently, "What are you feeding her now?"

"Oh, I am feeding her regular dog food now." I was so frustrated and upset that I went to the back of the building and sat down and looked at the wall for about ten minutes. "Father," I prayed, "if it's patience that I need to learn, then I will learn it."

I went back and told her very gently and kindly, "Let's get her back on her diet." She agreed and we did it. The dog straightened out again right away. But then the woman took ill and died. Her husband tried to continue the proper food, but he was old and ailing. The wife had cooked up enough food for several weeks ahead before she passed away. She knew she was dying. The old man brought the dog in a couple of times, but he couldn't cope. The last time he came in with his daughter, he had grown feeble to the point where he couldn't walk. The daughter made the decision to have the dog put to sleep.

We have slides of her last day. The girl brought her in and said she couldn't take care of her. "Dad is an invalid now and the dog is, too."

The little dog, at this point, was healthy and about fourteen or fifteen years old. I still have those slides, and in my imagination I can almost see that dog saying good bye.

I can still see the daughter, too. I can see the expression on her face, because she didn't want to do this. But she had to make a choice because she couldn't handle her father, either. Had they been eating macrobiotically, too, none of this would have been necessary.

I told her what I wanted to do. I wanted a record because I had taken slides through the years of the little dog. She consented to this. It was quite an emotional thing for me, too. This is especially true with an animal you have been treating for several years. Now I have assistants in the clinic. Most of the time when we have to have something like that done, we get the releases all signed. Then I walk to the back and I tell them to take care of it. I treat one dog now that is twenty-five years old. He's blind. And I have another that is around twenty. They have all benefited from macrobiotics. Becoming a macrobiotic veterinarian took me a while, but I could never turn back.

2
Growing Up in East Texas

My new found interest in natural healing took me back to my childhood and ancestral roots. I grew up on a farm in a corner of East Texas. It was thirteen miles to Clarksville, the nearest city, and thirteen miles to Idabell, Oklahoma. We lived in the sandy loam land before it dropped off into the alluvial soils that bottom out in the Red River.

My mother was a schoolteacher, and she taught us from an early age to seek knowledge and to read. To this day, I enjoy going to classes. I enjoy learning more. I feel that life itself is a school, and I feel that people evolve. You seek more knowledge and you reach a point called wisdom. My dedication is very simple. It's to improve the quality of life on planet earth, whether it be plant, animal, or human.

As I follow that and look for new things, I find that there is not anything really new under the sun. We just didn't see it. After getting into acupuncture and macrobiotics, I began to reflect on my life. I began to appreciate the traditional country way of life in which I was raised. I began to appreciate my ancestors, parents, and other relatives. I saw that to a great extent they lived in harmony with the natural world around them, especially with the plants and animals. In the deepest sense, they were macrobiotic. Only I had forgotten it when I went to school and veterinary college and became part of the modern world.

When I was eight, we moved to my grandmother's place. The farm covered about 300 acres. Originally there had been about 7500 acres in the homestead, located in different places and known by different names. There was the Bowe place and the Boudin place. These were named after the people the land had been bought from.

My grandmother was a great one for vegetables. She grew all kinds of vegetables and fruits. She would insist that we always eat vegetables at our meals. We had meat, but not so much. We ate grain as our principal food, especially cornmeal mush. Many a time that's what we would have for supper at night, just cornmeal mush. In the morning, if there was any left over, grandmother would fry that, and we would have it for breakfast. She also canned a lot. She had a big cellar and people always talked about how much food Mrs. Gentry had. She kept enough food in that cellar so that if nothing came up, we'd survive. We had a cellar full of canned vegetables, beans, and peas.

Our family ate them, especially in the winter. At other seasons, we also had potatoes and onions. We enjoyed apples from the orchards, and I carried one in my dinner bucket every day to school.

Every year they selected a beef. This was a traumatic time for me, because I didn't like to kill the animals. They let me have an old scrawny calf. His name was Shorty, and I raised him, worked with him, and even taught him to be ridden with a saddle. He grew into a big yearling. To me he was a pet, but naturally he was selected to become the beef. They killed him, and I never could take a bite of Shorty. I remember a man came over and helped Dad kill him. They knocked him in the head and cut his throat. I hid out behind the barn. I never did like to see the animals slaughtered. If there were extra cows to milk or somewhere to go like that, I managed to be gone if I could.

Dad always had hunting dogs, but I never enjoyed hunting. However, as a boy I was always called on to assist the older men. I had to carry the possums and coons that the men and dogs killed. I particularly didn't relish being out too late as I had to get up at four a.m. to build a fire and get ready to go to school.

But hunting was part of the way of life in East Texas at that time. Dad could get thirty dollars for a coon hide. That

15

was a lot of money in those days. We kept dogs just for hunting. They caught rabbits on their own, but most of all they loved squirrel. You could pick up a gun and act as if you were going squirrel hunting, and a rabbit would jump up right before the dogs and they would just look at him and let him run away. They weren't even interested. They loved to go squirrel hunting. I remember one day we killed fourteen squirrels. We went hunting on horseback, and they would join in the chase. We had a big squirrel stew and some people came over. We also had fried squirrel. The dogs ate the leftovers, including the insides and the hides.

The dogs just loved to go hunting. You could take a gun and make a sound like you were putting a shell in it, and they would go crazy. They also liked to hunt possums and raccoons and mink. You had to watch out for the coons, though. A smart old coon would get up on a log, and a dog would swim up to him and the coon would just take his front foot and put it over the dog's head and hold him under until he drowned. Smart dogs were aware of that and wouldn't swim out after a coon. Even here in Dallas, I had a client who lost eight dogs in one night to this coon.

Our dogs were primarily bluetick hounds and Walkers. We also had one redbone. Those are recognized breeds. We also had terriers—smooth-haired fox terriers. If you needed a cow put out of a pasture, you could call them. They did a good job of that. But the hounds wouldn't pay any attention to you. They were used for hunting. They didn't have any herding instinct at all. Terriers are quite helpful. When Daddy would be plowing, Bob—our terrier and the first dog I remember being attached to—thought it was his job to pull the trash away from the plow. He would just work like mad pulling cotton stalks away from the front of the plow. His tail was short and he was black with tan markings and he was one-eyed. He didn't weigh more than ten or twelve pounds. Today we would call him a Manchester.

One time Daddy took fifteen dollars and bought a bluetick hound. Momma was upset enough that he had spent all that money, but she was really upset when that dog got into some bread that was rising on the back porch. He got into it and ate the whole thing. There must have been three or four loaves. It hadn't been cooked yet and it was swelling. That dog began to swell up, too. I remember her saying, "I hope you bust!" Did she ever give Dad "Hail Columbia" about that dog eating up her bread.

Nothing was wasted. The saying was, down in that community, that the only thing that Mrs. Gentry lost in killing hogs or beef was the squeal or the bawl. She used everything else. We used to take the fat off the hides and render it up. We used it on our shoes to make them impervious to water. We also used it on the harnesses.

Despite his one eye, old Bob was a tough little guy. He ran out when he was a puppy and a big horse came by and he grabbed this horse by the heel. The horse kicked the eye out. One day a big dog came by, and Bob ran out and grabbed this big dog by his heel. The dog turned round and almost crushed his chest. We nursed him back to life, but he didn't want you to touch him. Any time you did, you got bitten.

There was a doctor in town who gave Dad a little old white dog. She was white and had one black ear and a black eye, and you couldn't get her to run cattle or anything. She would just sit there. But Bob taught her. Her name was Fannie. When she came into heat, we bred her to Bob. She had several litters, and we would give people puppies from her. She became a very brilliant dog owing to Bob. I used to get so tickled at watching them hunt rabbits together. Bob was a squirrel dog, and he wouldn't hunt rabbits at all. But if he was by himself or with Fannie, he'd take out after that rabbit and run it in a brush pile. The way they used to catch rabbits was interesting to watch.

How they learned this I don't know, but Bob would get on top of a brush pile and jump up and down until the rabbit came out. Fannie would take out after him, and the rabbit would run in a circle. Instead of running after them, Bob would run in the opposite direction. Many times he caught a rabbit. It would run right into his mouth. They would tear the rabbit open and eat the intestines. I always noticed that. That was where the plant matter was located. That was always the first thing they ate. Then if there was anything left, Fannie would take it and drag it. She'd dig a hole and bury it and dig it up and eat it a few days later. This was like partial cooking.

We kept Bob many years. One time we lost him and didn't know where he went. Dad said, "Bob would come home if somebody's not got him tied up, I know." One day we were going into town, driving an old Model T truck, and we saw Bob. A man had him in his wagon going along and had a log chain across the back. Bob was tied to this chain. Dad said, "That's old Bob. I know Bob." This was a real tough old man, known for knifing people. So Dad said, "I'll get some witnesses, and I am going to go get Bob." He got two men to go with him, and they drove down about ten to twelve miles where this man lived. Bob was in the yard, fenced up. Dad opened the gate, and Bob ran and got in the pickup behind the seat where he liked to ride. He liked to ride behind Dad's head. But you dared not reach your hand back there to touch him. He'd bite you.

Dad said, "Mr. Richardson, you got my dog. I come to get him." This man started cussing and said, "No, he wasn't either." The other fellows said, "Yeah, this is Mr. Ralston's dog. We know him." Dad said, "I'll tell you, Mr. Richardson. You say he is your dog. He's up behind the seat of that truck. If you can get him out of there without him biting you, you can have him." That old man wouldn't reach up there and get him, so we brought him home. Old Bob knew where he belonged.

We had another litter of puppies. We kept one called Little Joe, and he learned to hunt with Bob and Fannie. Money was tight so finally so one day this fellow came along and offered twenty dollars for Little Joe. Twenty dollars back in those days was a lot of money, and this guy wanted a good squirrel dog. Dad said, "That's a good one right there. I guarantee he will tree squirrels." The man bought him and took him up to Oklahoma. We were all attached to our animals, and the whole family was sad when Little Joe left. Everyone missed him. Then, guess what, that dog came home. He came back. He got away from those people in Oklahoma and came home. The pads on his feet were worn off. They were so sore he could hardly walk. But he came all the way back home, and so Dad said, "I'm not going to let him have him back. If he comes, I'll give him his money back. I'm not going to sell Little Joe, because he wants to stay here." The dog must have traveled at least fifty miles. He had to cross the Red River between Oklahoma and Texas to come home. We kept him until he died.

When we moved in with my grandmother, I entered school in a little one-room schoolhouse in a community called Vesey. We sat on long benches. If someone was against the wall and needed to get out, everybody had to get up and let the person out. About five sat on a row. Of course, there weren't very many students.

I went to that school until the sixth grade. Then I transferred to another school in Hopewell. We had to ride horseback because it was about three miles, including a mile over level land we called the flats. The flats were mostly covered with water. The other sections were solid woods. And was that flat section ever mosquitoey! I used to tell people, "I was raised where mosquitos were invented." It didn't take too long to ride, but the problem was that the horse made tracks in the mud and would step in a hole that had been stepped in before. The water then would shoot back, getting us all wet. When the weather was real bad, I'd wear a slicker. And sometimes it was so cold, the slicker would freeze to the horse.

The new school had two teachers. It was bigger and better, and Miss Cole was the principal. She was a good coach and put on two plays every year. One involved the students and the other, the people of the community. Of course, back in those days they didn't have television. Three or four hundred people would come from miles around to watch. That was one of the few entertainments we had. Folks would stand up outside. They didn't have seats. If rain came, the play would be canceled. We used bed sheets as backdrops. One time we put on a play under a church arbor. It had a big roof on it. I seemed to gravitate to the main part in the play. I played a porter. It was a comedy role, and I will never forget it. A train would be coming, and I would call out the names of my family and other people I knew.

The nearest high school was in Demple, thirteen miles

19

away. The bus didn't make it all the way to our farm, so I fixed a stable about three miles away. My Daddy helped me, and we put our horses in the stable and caught the bus from there. It was an old Model T bus. A fellow named Leatherwood drove it, and he would put us up at the stable and drive up to Demple. If you didn't get to the bus stop in time, you had to ride all the way.

I had a pair of Choctaw ponies. My sisters rode one of them, and I rode the other. I liked to go to school, and the horses would run at a pretty good gallop. The ponies were tough and would ride all day if you let them. My Daddy warned me, "Boy, you can go to school, but you're not going to feed that horse out of my corn bins. That's for working horses on the farm." So I raised peas in between the corn, and I picked those in the summertime and put them in a feed bin and fed those to my ponies in the winter.

The peas were a lot like aduki beans. We used to call them Red Rippers down in East Texas. They are real strong. Recently, I called a seed man down in Athens, Texas, the black-eyed pea capital of the country, and asked him where I could find some. He said, "We will give you twelve dollars a pound for them. Anybody that's got any we will pay that much because they are rare." I found some in the freezer that I had saved a few years earlier. I planted them and they came up. Now I have three acres. They are much stronger than black-eyed peas. Horses fed on those peas developed tremendous stamina and could literally go at a gallop all day long.

Sometimes my pony would play tricks on me. One time she got away. Her bridle was off and she decided to play. She would run with the saddle on and stay just out of reach. I would almost catch up to her, and she would kick up her heels and spurt ahead. I had to follow her all the way home. But she wouldn't do that all the time. Other times she would come right back when I talked to her.

I also remember an old thoroughbred. She had been a racehorse and got her leg messed up, and Daddy got her for a broodmare. She straightened out her leg, and she started running again. All she knew was how to run. One night we had to go two miles through the woods to school. The schoolteacher was putting on a play for the school patrons, and we were practicing. Bernice, my oldest sister, and I both had parts, and we set off on the back of this old mare.

Dad had always cautioned us not to let her get her head down. If she got the bits she would run away, and you couldn't stop her. We started home that time, and suddenly the sky darkened, and it looked like a tornado cloud was coming up. The winds began to blow and the horse started to run. My sister and I hung on for dear life as best we could. She got the bits in her mouth and ran away from us. I couldn't stop her, and Bernice was sitting behind me. There was a wire gate up ahead that was closed. The horse was running as fast as she could go and hit the wire gate, broke it, and went through without breaking stride. She ran all the way through the woods over crooked dirt roads. I wondered many times how in the world we kept from getting killed. But that old mare didn't stop until she got home and stuck her head over the iron gate to the horse lot. Then she stopped. There's a mystery and a power there that to this day I don't fully understand, but which I was determined to learn further about.

3
Learning from
My Grandmother

My love for animals was nurtured living with my grandmother. She was my first teacher, a constant source of natural wisdom and understanding. We had several cats growing up. The one I remember best was a big yellow tomcat. He had fathered a lot of kittens in his time, but down the line Dad had neutered him. I think we just called him Tom. Grandmother referred to him as a ratter. He was a big cat and quite capable of catching great big rats and killing them.

Late one dark, rainy, misty, cold day, a wagon with a sheet on it and a bow pulled up in front of our house. Two black men got out and helped lift a sick woman from the wagon. They carried her down the front walk into the house. We had a concrete walk in front of the house out to the road, and they brought her into the front room and set her in Grandpa's rocking chair. That was astonishing, because back in those days black people always came to the back door, and they had never before come into the house.

But apparently some arrangement had been made in advance, and now they arrived and set her in this chair. Grandma wrapped her up in a big comforter. A comforter is different from a quilt in that it's made of wool as well as cotton. The sight of this woman in the chair, too, was a big shock because the chair was almost sacred. Grandpa had been dead about twenty years, but his rocker was always a place of honor in the living room. Grandma always kept it in the same place. You could move every stick of furniture in the house and she wouldn't say a word, but you didn't fool with that chair.

The woman was very, very sick. After setting her down and making her comfortable, Grandma said to me, "Boy, go to the barn and bring me that old ratter." I went to the barn and got the cat and brought him back to the house. Grandma took the big orange cat and placed him on the woman's lap. She held her hands on it and told the woman to hold and stroke him, which she did all night long.

I was little, only about eight at the time, so I went to bed early. But the next morning, the sick woman got up and walked out to the wagon which had come back to fetch her. She was weak but able to walk. That amazed me, because so far as I could tell all Grandma had done was have her hold old Tom. "You are going to be all right now," Grandma told her as she got up in the wagon.

Many years later, after I got into acupuncture and macrobiotics, I began to understand what Grandma had done. She had put the cat over the lady's *hara*—the energy center deep in the intestines. She had the woman rub the cat to supply *ki*, or natural electromagnetic energy. When you rub your fingers or a comb along the back of a cat in the dark, you can see electricity spark there. Grandma was making an electrical circuit and feeding that energy into the *hara*. This is the area known in the Orient as the origin of life. That cat was a healthy cat, and the woman was picking up some of its *ki*. Since the meridians start or end in the fingers, by rubbing the cat, she was stimulating the *ki* flow down the meridians.

I told this experience in veterinary school, and I got laughed out of the class. I used to think that everything Grandma did was all right. I had thought all I had to do was get into veterinary school and that I knew everything. Then they laughed at me. It took me fifty years to appreciate her again.

Grandma had many home remedies. For instance, she taught us to harvest snake shed. That's the skin that a snake periodically sheds off. She kept a whole drawer full of them. On the farm, you would be walking along and you would see one, pick it up, and save it. Grandma used them for healing. She would take one out, put it in hot water, and then put it on the injured place. Say, for example, it was a splinter. She'd wrap it up at night with that snake shed. The next morning the splinter would be pulled to the surface. She used it on both people and animals for drawing out things and draining festers.

For poultices, she used peach tree leaves. She would mix them with cornmeal and put that on something that needed to be drawn out. She taught me that sassafras leaves are very good for relieving aching and pain. You can bruise the sassafras leaves, put them on the sore spot, and make a kind of covering over them, and it will give a lot of relief. They are very soothing.

She also used pine needles. She would bruise and beat them with a hammer. Then she put them in some water on the stove and turned it off just as it reached the boiling point. Then she would mix in a little oil and use the potion on a swollen leg or part. She would take the resin and put it on a cloth. It would be real stiff, and then she would apply it to the hurt spot. She used it to treat horses with colic. I remember she had me mix kerosene and pine resin together and hold it up to the horse's belly with the lid of a shortening bucket. The liquid would go away, and I always wondered where it went. She also made a lineament out of the resin. Later, when I studied Oriental medicine, I found they used the navel as an entryway into the body. She knew that! It was amazing.

Grandma also used salt and epsom salt. She would take epsom salt, put it between two layers of cloth, and wrap it around a limb. To stop something from bleeding, she would go to the stovepipe and get soot. She would put it on the cut, and it would stop. Once a horse had a bad cut and was bleeding profusely. Grandma took a bunch of soot, put it on a cloth, and placed it on the wound. It stopped in no time. Old-fashioned dentists often use soot in the form of creosote to stop bleeding, too.

When we were fattening hogs, she would mix in burned charcoal with their feed. She said it made them digest their food better. I noticed it seemed to work.

One time a fellow who was working for us got a thorn in his leg. His ankle swelled up to two to three times its normal size. She had him soak it in a bucket with warm water and salt. It got better. She always seemed to know something to do for minor injuries like that. Someone would always come and ask her, "Well, what can you do?" And she would say, "Let's do this." White people, black people, country people, city people—everyone came, and she helped them all.

She grew a lot of plants and herbs in her garden. She made teas out of the leaves and vines and had the person drink them. She used asparagus, for example, as a diuretic. If someone had a problem with urination, she gave them asparagus tea.

I never saw a sick cat in my life on the farm. They were healthy and had a variety of things to eat. The dogs were healthy, too, though they could be bitten by a snake, and Grandma would make a poultice for that. She always gave the cats cow's milk whenever there was a new calf. That milk contains colostrum in it and is highly nutritious. She didn't feed them a lot, but she fed them some every day. "You don't want to feed them too much," she would say, "or they'll get lazy. You want them to be hunting." I remember her sitting and watching this rabbit that was getting in the garden and getting her vegetables. She said to one mother cat she had, "Now you go catch that old rabbit." Sure enough, that cat sat for hours waiting for the rabbit to come, and she got it.

Grandma had one old cow that used to challenge her. Her name was Polly. She was the worst kicker we had on the place. I have seen that cow knock her down and kick her under the sill of the barn. Grandmother would put a strap on Polly's leg with a ring in it and tie a rope on to keep Polly from kicking her. Polly seemed to know. Whenever it was on, she wouldn't kick, but as sure as Grandmother left it off, Polly would wham her. They had a real contest going.

Another time a chicken snake got into the hen nest and took the eggs. Grandma took Fannie, one of our dogs, and went out there and put her in the chicken house. She said, "She'll get that rascal." Next day, Fannie had killed that snake.

When Grandma went to the barn, the cats always greeted her. The cats she kept in the cow barn didn't go into the horse barn. And the one in the horse barn didn't go into the cow barn. Sometimes she would make gravy for the cats. She would take some bacon or meat fixings and then add flour and milk and give them some. There was no such thing as cat food then. I never saw cat or dog food until I was grown. She would give them a variety of things. She even gave the cats cooked carrots. She would mix them in the gravy.

We had another big ratter who lived in the horse barn. When you went into the corn crib, he liked to go in there with you. I would go in there and move the corn around, and I would see him leap and grab a mouse or rat in nothing flat. I don't know how high he leapt, but it was amazing. He knew when you moved that corn around, a mouse was liable to come out. He would be ready and sit right there with you. I would move something and if I heard a noise, I'd say in a half whisper, "Listen, listen. He's right there. Listen." He would jump and grab the mouse when it appeared. He was very accurate.

We had rats, too. Some of them were pretty good sized. But this old cat could kill any rat. These rodents would eat the corn if they could. I remember one time Grandma was saving seed corn. She would shell it and pick out the best grains to plant. There was a sack she kept to put these grains in for planting. One day a rat cut a hole in it, and the corn began leaking out. About a half gallon was lost, and she said, "We'll get that scalewag." She got the cat and put him in the corn crib and shut the door. "He'll get him tonight," she said. "He'll come back." And sure enough, the next day, he killed that rat, and there was hardly any evidence where he had killed and eaten him.

In addition to corn, the mice and rats ate cottonseed meal and peas. But they didn't like peas nearly so much as ground corn. They just loved corn. That was one of the reasons I liked to have peas around. They wouldn't mess much with the peas. But you had to be careful and keep them under control or they would destroy a crib of corn. That was the cats' job, and we didn't have any problem.

Of course, we ate the corn, too. We took it to the mill back in those days. We would shell the corn and save the good kernels for Grandma's sack. We finally got a corn sheller of our own. You put an ear of corn in it and turned a crank, and it shelled the corn. But Grandma didn't much like the machine because all the bad kernels got in with the good ones, and she'd have to go through and pick them out. It was really easier to shell it by hand. At the end of the cob, there would be little undeveloped grains. She didn't want those in with the seed corn.

We didn't have bread on the farm. Sometimes she would send me with a sack of shelled corn across my pony's back to the grist mill about six miles away. Mr. Jackson operated the mill, and we'd either pay or give him a third of the corn to grind it. He'd put the remaining two thirds back in the sack. We used to call these crocus sacks. Most of the time I'd ride bareback when I went to the mill. It was more comfortable than riding with a saddle. Then I'd come back and give Grandma the cornmeal, and she would fix corn bread. Now that was what you'd call good, fresh corn bread.

Grandma had a Willey's Overland. It was a little car and not very dependable. Of course she also had a buggy, one we called a hack. Two horses pulled it, and she used it a lot. The hack was an easy way to travel because it was light, and the horses trot a lot and travel faster. It wasn't like pulling a heavy wagon. In 1934 she bought a new Chevrolet.

Several years before that time, they came out with the first radio. I never will forget when we first went to hear the radio. A fellow named Tom Mosley had one. We would go over to his house on Saturday night and take turns listening with earphones. You had to wear them to keep down the static. Sometimes you couldn't get the signal at all. Then our family got a radio. They had improved them, and we thought it was so pretty. We went out in the woods, found a big tall pine, ran an aerial up this tree, and played the radio with the car battery. The only problem was that you could only play it one day. Then the battery would be so low that you would have to take it back to town and have it charged up so you could hear the radio again.

Grandma bought this new Chevy with a radio, and it was terrific. You could hear the Grand Ole Opry and the National Barn Dance and programs like that. But we almost killed ourselves listening to that thing. Bernice, my oldest sister, and Edwina, my younger sister, and I would slip out to the garage to listen to the radio. We kept the garage door closed because we didn't want anyone to know that we were listening to the radio and running the battery down. The only thing that saved us from asphyxiation was that the garage door wouldn't close completely. There was a big crack, and the exhaust from the motor must have gone outside. It was a miracle we weren't killed.

Grandma also kept cats in the smokehouse. That was where the meat was kept. It was built over a cellar in the ground. She had built this a long time before we came to live with her. She stored food that needed refrigeration down in the cellar and kept the meat in the smokehouse above. The meat was kept on a string on a wire so the mice couldn't get at it. But she kept a cat in that area, and the cat that stayed there she called a house cat, and it came in on the back porch. She would take it in the house some, but she controlled that too. She managed all the cats herself.

Our family fared fairly well through the Great Depression. We lived on about five dollars a week. When I was about twelve or thirteen, they needed somebody over at the sawmill to pull the sawdust away from the mill. My Daddy hired out the team of horses and me for $2.50 a day—two dollars for the team and fifty cents for me. He assured the man that I could handle it. I was pretty good at driving the team.

Compared to other families, we made it through the Depression years very well. Grandma saw that we had enough to eat. I would hear people say, "Why, I bet old Lady Gentry's got enough canned goods in that cellar over there to last two or three years, if she didn't take no crop at all." And she probably did. We ate what we raised and raised what we ate.

I had one pair of overalls that I wore to school. My instructions were always to take my school clothes off when I came home. That was the first thing you did when you came home from school: you put on raggedy clothes. They had a lot of patches, and I remember one time Momma saying, "We got more patches than we got cloth."

My mother saved every scrap of cloth there was and pieced them together in a quilt. If you didn't have anything to do, she'd teach you to quilt. She'd say, "An idle mind is the devil's workshop. I'll give you something to do." She would have you in there quilting. I learned to quilt that way. The quilting frame could be pulled up to the ceiling and kept out of the way or it could be let down to work on. Before long, you would have a new quilt.

Every bit of time was utilized like that. This was the one objection I had growing up: I always felt that I didn't have enough time to play. Now, after a half century of living as an adult in the modern world, I miss those early, carefree years on the farm—even the work. But then modern agriculture bears almost no resemblance to the traditional farm on which I grew up.

4

From the Family Farm to the Factory Farm

I grew up in close contact with animals, and I remember them as though they were members of my family. When I was a young boy, my father gave me a little pig of my own. I had just got to where she knew me, and I heard about a terrible outbreak of cholera that was spreading through the county. Back in those days, hogs ran "outside," meaning there were no fences and everybody's hogs ran together. You told which hogs were yours by notches that you cut in their ears when they were babies. Each person had their own ear marks.

Hogs were dying all over the place, and I was worried sick that my little pig would get cholera. I finally figured out a way to isolate her. There was an old vacant barn on my grandmother's farm that was about a half mile from the house. The barn had two good stables and a fence that completely surrounded it. I slipped my pig up there, put her in one of the stables, closed the door. Then I repaired the lot fence so that no hog could come near her.

I had no trouble getting my little pig to follow me to the barn. She had already learned that she was special to me because I would cut her out of the herd and give her a little extra corn or peas. I just offered her a little corn, and she followed me like a puppy.

Now that I had her isolated I had to go there every morning to feed her. Every morning at 4:00 A.M., I fed her regardless of the weather. Facing the north wind carrying a kerosene lantern and a bucket of feed was quite a challenge for a small boy. I remember the more I cared for her, the more attached we became. We talked a lot as I fed and rubbed her each morning. I couldn't bear the idea that she might some day be killed for people to eat. I named her Dixie.

The cholera came, and Daddy lost hogs by the droves. They would bed down together at night, and the next morning they would all be dead. They were stacked together one on top of the other like pieces of firewood. My father lost every hog he had. Not one survived. We burned every last one to ashes. Dixie was the only hog to survive the epidemic.

Spring finally came, and Dixie had grown into quite a young gilt. My grandmother said, "It's time Dixie goes a courtin'." She came into heat, and I fashioned a crate out of some boards and put them on a wooden sled. I put Dixie in the crate, hitched a mule to the sled, and set out for a neighbor's place about five miles away. He had a nice male hog and insisted that I leave her so they could get acquainted. That meant that the mule and I would have to make two trips with that sled, but that was all right because Dixie was getting bred, and she was a fine hog.

My grandmother taught me that the pregnancy is a very important time. She told me that the mother needed special care during that period because she was building babies inside her body. I wanted Dixie to have the best, so I listened very carefully.

I watched her every day as she got bigger and bigger. I depended on my grandmother for advice. It was a very exciting time for me, watching her build a bed in which to have the babies. My grandmother had me provide her with a lot of clean pine straw that I gathered in the woods. Finally the labor started. She had nine piglets, all healthy and hungry. I was there as each one came out, talking to her and reassuring her but not interfering. There were eight little girls and one little boy. Dixie was a great mother, and all nine pigs survived.

My father was impoverished from his loss, so I gave him all the females, and they became his brood sows. The male I gave to the neighbor, for I owed him a pig for the breeding service. It was thrilling to watch Dixie's offspring as they developed, and I had the satisfaction of helping my father get back into the hog business.

There was always activity and the excitement of new life on the farm. The dogs would all bark whenever somebody came. We didn't have a lot of company. Sometimes people who came were lost and needed directions. Then there would be the peddlers with their wares. They always carried a chicken coop on their backs. Grandmother would trade chickens for different things they had, such as vanilla extract. She loved vanilla extract. There wasn't very much money.

We never tied up or leashed a dog, unless it was a female in heat. If Daddy didn't want Fanny to get bred, he would put her in the corn crib. He would keep her in there until she went out of heat. Grandmother knew how to take care of the females when they were pregnant. She would tell me, "Always keep a smile on the face of a pregnant girl." She put that principle to work everywhere. She felt the pregnant female cat, dog, horse, cow, or hog should have extra care. When Dixie, my horse, was pregnant, she had me getting up at four a.m. and going a half mile to the barn with two buckets of extra food and water and a couple of ears of corn in my back pocket.

The dogs ate out in the backyard and had their own bowl. The cats never seemed to bother it. The cats fended for themselves. We didn't have an overpopulation of cats, as you might think. They weren't spayed or castrated as a rule. The hounds would kill baby kittens. You had to watch out for them. One time they killed a litter and Grandma said, "If they are going to be doing that, they are going to have to leave." Dad said, "We'll see that they don't get in here anymore."

When I was nine years old, Dad took me up to Millertown, Oklahoma, to a place where they castrated mules and calves. I learned how to do that. Interestingly, our farm animals never had infections. We washed them off with water, but didn't have any disinfectant or chemicals. I remember them talking about castrating a dog or cat, but I never saw my Daddy do it. Usually they just shut up the females in the barn. I never saw a dog castrated until I was in college.

Except in wealthy homes where they were kept as special pets, dogs and cats and other animals were always part of the natural environment. Dogs worked and had a purpose. I remember my grandfather buying two hounds. They were redbone, and he named them Drum and Bugle. Old Bugle got run over by a hay rake and was killed, and you could hear Old Drum mourn. It was quite thrilling to go hunting with dogs like that and listen to them run. By the way they barked, you could tell what they were doing. There is a special bark when they tree an animal. Today, people are far removed from the cycles of life and death. But in those days, the times were hard and people were abandoning farms. There was no work and folks would just leave the country with what they had. I have seen them put everything they had on an old Model T Ford and take off and leave the cats behind. Normally you would expect the place to be run over with cats, but they wouldn't be. Three or four cats would survive. I found out by watching them. The male cat would kill the baby kittens and any cats that came around. Anything that threatened his kingdom was killed off. There wouldn't be fifteen or twenty cats as you might expect. That's part of the way nature has of keeping the population down. There seems to be a rhythmic balance and interchange in nature.

In contrast to the traditional family farm, modern farming puts the animals under tremendous stress. I think it's terrible. I am more of a vegetarian now, but if I ate meat I would never touch anything that had been raised like that. The animal raised under stress will transmit that stress to the person who eats the meat.

The U.S. Department of Agriculture sponsors a lot of chemicals and sprays. Recently, I was down at my brother-in-law's in Clarksville. A beautiful pair of oak trees used to mark his place where you turn in the gate. I would always watch for those trees as I drove up. The first thing I noticed on my last visit was that the two trees were dead. It takes seventy-five years for trees to grow to that size.

There also used to be a beautiful pair of shade trees in the backyard that kids played under. Both were dead. Then my brother-in-law told me that he had been having this chronic headache. His head hurt something awful. He had tried different things, and even went to an acupuncturist I recommended, which helped some. I asked him if he had been using chemicals on his spread. He said, "I sprayed up there. That could have killed those trees." I inspected his cows and found they had big tags in their ears recording the insecticides used on them. That challenges the liver day and night.

He didn't know why the two trees in the backyard died, but I knew why. Where did he think he was getting his headache from? My sister's had some problems too, and she's got two little grandchildren she's raising. People like this have been controlled for years by folks at the U.S.D.A. and the county agents. And who are *they* controlled by? The fertilizer and chemical industries.

I had a friend who was an agriculture teacher in a town east of Clarksville and he had a son. His son went to Texas A&M and ended up teaching in a small place called Siegleville. I sent him word that I'd known his papa and would like to see him. I mentioned organic farming. He had never heard of it. This was a man with a master's degree in agriculture. It's incredible.

They teach them to run a tractor, how to weld and do a lot of technical things. But as for the basics—organic farming and taking care of planet earth—they are woefully ignorant.

Factory farming is producing more for less, at least that's the theory. But it's also been sponsored by the people who are interested in selling their product. They teach and tell the public that it is in their interest to do thus and so. But I feel this is exploitation.

The American farmer is one of the most exploited people on the earth. He has been exploited by the fertilizer companies and the chemical companies. Now we've got to pay the price; they have contaminated our environment. I used to love to drive in the spring to see the beautiful flowers. Then they started spraying, and you have to keep the windows up in the car. You hit valleys where there is so much insecticide you can hardly breathe. I will never forget when they came out with DDT. "It's absolutely harmless, Doctor," the fellow selling it assured me, mixing it with his hands. "Houses in the future will not be built with screens because they won't need them. All you do is spray with this stuff and no more insects."

They went out through the country spraying everybody's houses. I thought at the time, "Hey, this is not right." That was a good many years ago. Of course, they have taken DDT off the market now, but the birds and insects are still affected. Take the horned toad. In this area, he was a little guy that used to eat the insects. Now he's extinct. I haven't seen him in ten years. So as I looked at my brother-in-law's home, I said, "A farm should reflect life, and it reflects death." It scares me, and I can't say that enough.

The man who owns the land next to mine has promised that I can buy it when he gets ready to sell. He didn't tell me he was going to clear-cut. He clear-cut it and sprayed it, and I can't stand to go there anymore. I just cried when I found out. There were trees over a hundred and fifty years old that were sprayed and cut down. I hate it. One time in Arkansas I climbed a fire tower, and as far as I could see, the land had been clear cut. I was on my way to Broken Bow, Oklahoma, and above Broken Bow I had this terrible headache. I couldn't bear the smell and odor. I found out they had sprayed the whole county. Later there was an article in the paper reporting that a lot of women were miscarrying and having children with birth defects from all this spraying.

They call that tree farming, but that's factory farming. The same thing is happening with the animals. They're giving them antibiotics that are poisoning and weakening them. And they're enrolling veterinarians to test and administer these chemicals. It's amazing but true that most veterinary schools still don't have a nutrition program. There are only one or two around the country that do. They have no idea what a balanced diet is. The commercial interests have exploited the veterinarian as they have exploited the farmer. This is one of the reasons I won't talk to drug salesmen anymore. We still buy some drugs, but I make someone else do that. Then I look at the order and either okay it or turn it down. I know all their tricks.

When I moved to Dallas in 1955, they began giving tetracycline to chickens. At slaughter, they dipped them in this antibiotic and then packaged them. It was supposed to give them a long life. The chicken turned bitter, and then they injected diethylsilbesterol in the chicken's neck. That's now better known as DES—a major cancer-causing chemical that causes birth defects in humans. I said, "No way am I going to do that." It took until 1980 to stop that practice. Then when the results of that became known, they took the chicken necks and put them in the dog food. The dog breeders finally sued to make them stop. All their females went sterile, and they traced it back to the DES.

A lot more suits like that need to be filed. I think we need a class action suit against the companies that make tetracycline. A lot of people and animals have had damage done to their livers because of that antibiotic. The companies knew the effects but continued to sell it. I had a herd of registered Angus down in East Texas and naturally got involved in the politics of cattle exhibition. First, they would go in and cut what they called ties in their backs. They would take a knife and cut the hide loose to form an even top line. The fat would push up and the hide would be attached and that would make a little dent, so they wanted to cut those so it would make a smoother top line. I was told I would have to do this if I wanted to win. You were also supposed to take a big tube, about two inches in diameter, push it down the show cow's mouth, and force feed it to make it gain weight. This is when I quit showing registered cattle completely. I said, "Forget it, Charlie. If that is what it takes, God forbid I should ever be involved."

Fortunately, there is some common sense and decency left. I heard about one man who was having problems selling his cattle, so he decided he'd go organic like Frank Ford out in Hereford, Texas. Frank had to build houses in the winter to make a living and get Arrowhead Mills off the ground: they used to laugh at him when he went down to Texas A&M. "There goes that old organic farmer." Now Arrowhead Mills is extremely successful, and they roll out the red carpet for him.

If a person signs up with a farm to go into his program, they have to wait three years while they clean up the soil and get the chemicals out. But Frank pays them premium for their grain, and they want that good market. People are beginning to see the light, thank God. You have to respect nature, or in the end it will do you in. If you respect nature and work with it, it will produce the best.

Not long ago, I went to a feed store I used to frequent. I loved to go in there and just smell the fresh grain and the grinding corn. But I wouldn't work there now for a million dollars a day. The woman behind the counter couldn't stop talking about her allergies. The odor of the insecticides was so strong I could hardly breathe. I didn't say one word; I just walked out.

5
The Human-Animal Bond

Over the years, in my life as a husband, father, veterinarian, and citizen of the community, I have found that love is the attracting, uniting force in our universe. Nowhere is this uniting force better demonstrated than between man and his animals. Only the bonding force between mother and child is as strong. Sometimes an animal serves as a substitute for the mother-child love bond. This is well demonstrated by the breeds of small dogs that serve as baby substitutes for many people. The truest expression of love has been described as the complete giving of oneself, with no expectation of anything in return. This is perfectly demonstrated in societies where, although starvation is present, many will share their meager fare with their animals. Older people in the direst of circumstances, too, will feed and provide for their animals in preference to improving their own lot.

I recall an elderly woman who I first met when she started bringing a very old cat to me. As time went by and I became acquainted with her family of animals, I found that her pets ranged from cats and dogs to chickens and a very old turkey gobbler. For many years she paid her bill in cash carried in a small Bull Durham tobacco sack, which she kept hidden under her skirt or in her slacks and secured with a safety pin. She would excuse herself, turn away from you, reach up under there, and take out the money to pay the bill. I recognized that her circumstances were at least very moderate, and her bill was always kept to the bare minimum. Our business relationship had gone on for over fifteen years when I noticed that her visits had almost stopped, and that she would have a friend call to inquire about the price of some service.

At this point I decided to do a little investigation. I discovered an appalling situation. The man she had worked for had died. She lived in a little two-room shack beside what had been his house. There was running water, but no hot water. Her total income was sixty-three dollars per month from Social Security. She had survived the previous winter on what she could garner from garbage cans behind a local grocery store and an occasional fried chicken dinner that an employee from a massage parlor next door shared with her.

Needless to say, I charged her not one penny from that day forward for the veterinary care of her animals. I also contacted the local welfare office head, who happened to be a good friend, and asked that her circumstances be investigated. She was furious with me! She would not allow the case worker on the place. Her biggest fear was that she would be placed in a nursing home and her "little darlings" would be destroyed. Much coaxing and persuasion finally convinced her that nothing was going to be done to her. She accepted welfare help and food stamps, and her circumstances improved considerably.

Though her existence seemed almost beyond human endurance, not one of her pets could be called neglected. Her love for her animals, and theirs for her, followed her to the grave. She was killed one day crossing the freeway on one of her many trips to the grocery store—probably to get food for her pets. She was eighty-nine. Even though her life was snuffed out suddenly, I know she died happy because she had the animals she loved to the very end.

The story does not end there! Friends who knew her took the responsibility of looking after her pets—and I still treat them for free. The old turkey gobbler is approaching eighteen years.

The purpose of telling this story is to demonstrate the strong bond between humans and their animals. Many other stories could be told of such a bond—a bond of love. On the other side of the fence, animals, especially dogs, have demonstrated their love for their masters many times. One I recall vividly from my childhood concerns our family dog, Bob. Old Bob went with us everywhere. One of our favorite things that my cousins and I did was to slip off from our folks and go swimming. We would go to the stock tank or a swimming hole in the nearby creek. My mother was deathly afraid of snakes and forbid us to go there, because it was full of cottonmouth water moccasins. Bob seemed to feel it was his duty to protect us. When he knew we were heading for the swimming hole, he would creep up to the water, and when he spotted a snake, he would dive in, swim underwater, and grab the snake in his mouth, swim to shore, and kill the snake. Bob hated snakes, and he seemed compelled to protect mischievous boys. I had seen his head swollen to twice his body size from a battle with a rattler, and his hatred of snakes finally did him in. He was bitten in his only good eye by a copperhead one day as we built fences, and he died before we could get him home to Grandma for treatment. We were very sad, of course. We knew he had died in his effort to save us. We knew he had loved us, and we had loved him. My memory of him is one of my treasures.

The medical community is now beginning to recognize the importance of the love that we share with our animals. The bond between animals and humans is important for normal development. Through the years, I have observed that the animal abusers tend to be child abusers. But animals can even help change cruel people to kind ones.

Take the case of Mr. A., who came to work for me when I was in desperate need of kennel help. At the time, we were doing a lot of bathing, clipping, and grooming of dogs. Mr. A. was a typical cotton farmer who had moved to the city when cotton farming failed, and he tried to survive by seeking a job. He had a slight case of Parkinson's disease, which caused the involuntary shaking of his hands. He was in his late fifties and had been seeking work for several months. He seemed honest and desperately needed a job, so I hired him. But while doing routine kennel work, he was severely bitten or clawed fourteen times in the first ten days. After a particularly nasty bout where he was severely bitten, I fired him. After he left, my receptionist remarked that she hated to see Mr. A. go because he desperately needed a job, and she proceeded to relate to me the state of his home life. His wife of many years had a serious mental sickness that was incurable and was in desperate need of institutional care. Mr. A. had sought help for her but due to his ignorance and desperate financial situation, he had been unable to get proper support. Her condition was so severe that he was unable to get the rest he needed at home.

I called him back to work. Before I would allow him to start, I sat him down for a long counseling session. I explained to him that working with animals could be a joy. I wrote the name of every animal in big, bold letters and attached the name to every cage. He was instructed to greet each dog or cat by name every time he came near the cage. He was taught to take the animals out of their cages, stroke them, and speak in a low voice.

I expected improvement, but I was amazed at the transformation that continued until the end of Mr. A.'s days. He became so proficient in handling animals that just his presence in the kennel would calm a distraught animal. He became a real genius at handling both dogs and cats. We got institutional care for his wife, and he learned that the love and tenderness he gave to the animals was returned tenfold.

We boarded lots of animals then, and many times I saw regular boarders leave their owners and run back to the kennel to see Mr. A. He always spoke to the animal first when people brought their pets in.

So there is hope even for people who seem cruel and indifferent. The bottom line is love. I believe that the cruel person is expressing his or her need for love. Of course the animals need to be ensured of safety, but I feel the use of animals in helping solve social problems offers great hope.

Here in Dallas, a little girl was inspired by a puppy to get well. She had an accident that left her ninety-two percent of her body burned. The child refused to eat and yet needed three times the ordinary amount of food due to the excessive demand of her badly burned body for nutrients. Finally, the promise of a puppy inspired her to take the food that she needed for the healing to take place. The puppy was brought to the hospital and continued to strengthen the girl's will to live. According to the report I saw, the puppy was washed, wrapped in a sheet, and slipped into the hospital against regulations. This is another beautiful example of the human-animal bond of love.

During my food trials at the clinic, the animals I cooked for seemed happier and more energetic, and their hair coats became shinier. Even one that had heartworms improved in both coat and attitude. This evidence helped me in formulating the treatment that I now use. The animals began to smell better, their breaths smelled clean, and their stools were not too offensive.

Inevitably, close ties developed between me and the animals I was caring for. I recall one dog in particular. He was black, part Labrador in ancestry, and of course I called him Blackie. I took him from an owner who could no longer keep him. In doing routine tests, I found that he had heartworm. Since I was already involved in feeding trials, I decided to put him in the group. I kept him in the test group for about two and one-half years, all the while feeding him an excellent diet, observing him daily, and retesting about every two weeks. He responded to good nutrition better than I had expected. I gave him the treatment that I had worked out for heartworm, and in thirty days he showed a clear test. He had a beautiful shiny coat, was active, and had tested negative to repeated heart worm tests over a period of about a year and a half.

I was really attached to the guy. He loved water and would swim out and retrieve things that I threw. One day I got to thinking it was a shame that a dog that liked the outdoors so much did not have a farm to run on and a lake to swim in. About that time, an older gentleman came in and expressed interest in finding a larger dog. He said that he had a farm with a small lake about fifty miles away, that he planned to retire there in the next month or so, and that he would like to have a dog for a companion. I introduced him to Blackie and they were an immediate pair. With a mixture of sadness and joy, I told Blackie good bye. They came back for annual checkups for several years, but now both owner and dog have passed on.

I could tell many stories like this. Recently, a nurse who was doing private duty for a man with a serious heart condition brought in a Chihuahua puppy she had acquired for him. She told me that she could not believe the improvement she has seen in the man since the puppy arrived on the scene.

Another person deeply affected by the presence of an animal was an old woman in a nursing home. She was by herself and nobody could communicate with her. She would eat if someone took a spoon and put food into her mouth, but she would just sit by herself and could not socialize or talk to anyone. Now there was a Doberman pinscher at the nursing home who was owned by a physical therapist. They turned the dog loose, and he singled out this woman, lying his big old head in her lap. She began to pet him and told them that she wanted a dog. She started to communicate again, and every day they brought this dog to her and let her pet him. She gradually came out of her shell and got well. I have heard stories like this about children who have been helped by animals as well. A book called *The Four-Footed Therapist* relates the experiences of a woman who used a cat and a dog in different therapeutic situations.

Animal Rights

I am thankful that there is a growing awareness of animal rights. I am hopeful that as we evolve toward a more peaceful way of being we will have more respect for life. Recently, a leading university was fined and its research programs shut down and reorganized because of cruelty to animals in the laboratories. I admire the courage of the people who brought this to the attention of the public.

It grieves me to know that there are thousands of animals suffering at this very moment in research projects. I think it is time for us to speak out. It is time we stopped most of these so-called research projects that add little or nothing to our scientific knowledge. Confinement is cruel, especially confinement in an unnatural environment. Any information coming from research conducted using animals in such stressful conditions is information that I would hold highly suspect.

The cruel practice of selling unfortunate dogs and cats to scientific and medical centers needs to be addressed, too. I once heard a nationally respected veterinarian say, "We have enough misinformation on misinformation." I could not agree more. My prayer for those who commit this crime against animals is "Forgive them, Father, for they know not what they do."

The issue of humane euthanasia needs to be addressed, too. It is ridiculous to accept that one method is more humane than any other in all circumstances. The ideal method, of course, is where the animal is gently restrained, one of the quick-acting euthanasia products is given intravenously, and only the slight discomfort of a sharp needle is felt. On the other hand, if we are faced with the distasteful task of euthanizing a large number of fearful animals, to catch each one and restrain them so that they can be humanely given an intravenous injection can be downright cruel. Certainly this unpleasant task should be supervised by a doctor of veterinary medicine. However, he or she should be free to make the choice of method to use based on his or her judgment and experience. I have lived in the hope that the AVMA—the American Veterinarians Medical Association—would appoint a blue-ribbon committee to study the matter and come up with some common sense recommendations. However, getting our AVMA to take a stand is like getting a politician to say something definite.

I would like to share with you a simple prayer that I find helpful when I am faced with this distasteful responsibility, "Father, I commend the spirit of this thy creature into thy hands." A wonderful book for you to read is *Kinship of All Life*.

Animals as Our Weather Vanes

The way we treat animals is becoming more of an issue

worldwide, and I am encouraged, because the situation is so much better than it was. Holistic medicine is continuing to evolve, and we are going to understand that it's better for us to have healthy bodies. We are going to see that exploiting with drugs is not the way to go. How we treat animals is our weathervane.

I had a little cat in yesterday that had been through a lot of unnecessary surgery and was put through a lot of pain because of a tumor. There wasn't any sense in it. Gradually we are becoming aware of that, and the public, bless them, is ahead of many professionals. They are saying, "So you say this is clean food? What is this? What is that?"

Public attitudes about cruelty to animals have changed a lot. When I was just starting a practice here in Dallas, there was a place near my office that exercised horses. A man there was beating a horse, and when I tried to intervene, they threatened my life. They finally stopped, but I had to get away from there because I was about to get into real trouble. My family was with me, and I didn't want my children to hear all that stuff. But if such a thing were to happen today, I wouldn't have to say a word. Ten people would intervene. Back then, a whole group of people stood and watched while this man beat an animal for no reason at all, except that he had a bad temper. The horse didn't have a bad temper, the man did. That incident couldn't happen here today.

There are still abuses. Take rodeo, for instance. Now to me it is cruel to take an animal and repeatedly use it for roping, throwing it down on the ground. It doesn't understand, and after you have done that to it for several months, you send it off to the slaughterhouse.But gradually the situation is improving. Now they have breakaway roping. They rope the animal and break away, and that doesn't jerk the animal down. It's much more humane.

One time when I was running the Society for Animal Protection, a man came in and got a puppy. Because of his negligence, the puppy froze to death. I then taught him how to take care of an animal and let him have another. I was roundly criticized for that. To my way of thinking, it's much better to teach someone than to punish them. We should have video tapes and make them available to teach people how to take care of a puppy or kitten. Now somebody might say, "Everybody knows that, but you would be surprised at how many don't know.

Children especially need to be trained about the proper way to handle animals. I had a little Chihuahua in the other day that had been injured by a child. A little kid just picked this little dog up and threw it. The boy throws his toys, so he threw the puppy and broke its leg. I tried to talk to him and show him how to be gentle with animals. I think that is one of the responsibilities of my profession, as well as of all humane societies.

Actually, we are teaching love in this way. Take the exposure of older people to animals. Even some of the big dog food companies are seeing now that the aging person wants to get a pet. They have a program now where an elderly person can go to the SPCA to get a pet, and the food companies will even pay for some of the initial expenses. At my clinic, we are working out a program—a well-puppy program—in which we give the first exam free to get them started in the right way. There are little things we can teach people about taking care of their animals.

I have a rapport with animals that I gained as a child, and it's something that very few people have. I feel sorry for children who never have any pets, because I feel that giving and receiving love from animals is very important to human development.

Learning from Animals

We learn many things and develop many qualities from interacting with animals. We learn to respect another life form. My own little cousin was killed on my pony, Dolly, when I was eleven years old. Dolly stopped immediately when he fell off. He had been making her run, but when he fell, she stopped immediately. And a horse will teach you ways that he can escape you so that you will treat him properly. I used to try to ride my pony Pet. We had a very close relationship. I could take a corn shuck and rattle and call her, and she would come up to me. A lot of times I would just swing up on her back with no bridle or saddle and ride her like an Indian. But I didn't reward her or feed her, I would have a hard time catching her the next time. She taught me, "You've got to take care of me if you expect me to work for you." This was a very good experience for me.

We used to have certain cows to milk, and my mother had me go down to the barn to take some warm water to wash the cow's udder. If I didn't feed the cow and wash her udder, or didn't wait and let her relax, she might just wham me up the side of the head with her foot. That kick meant, "You know better than to treat me like that." This is the way that you learn.

Horses taught me they are much stronger than I am, so I have to respect their strength. Many people get hurt by a gentle animal, especially by a large animal like a horse or a cow. They get hurt because they don't respect the animal's strength. I will restrain an animal if an animal is trying to bite me; I will get rough, just as rough as it takes to restrain the animal. But then I try to let the animal know that I am not angry with it.

Some animals are remarkably intelligent. I used to have some little mules that I worked with, hauling this little wagon. I had to keep the harness aligned, because if a mule found he could turn his neck, which is very strong, he could slip out of the harness and run away. I had to watch that very closely. Now horses are not as smart as mules are. You go near one of those manhole covers in the street, and you can't make a mule step on one of those to save your life. He knows better. The thing might be loose, and his leg might go through and be hurt. But a horse might stick his foot through there and break his leg. If there is a hole in the bridge and he's walking across, a horse sometimes might stick his foot through there, but not a mule. A mule is always watching where he puts his feet. That's why they are such good animals in the mountains. They can climb great heights, watch where they put their feet.

Pigs, too, are real smart. They have ways of talking. A mama pig has a certain way she grunts to get all the little pigs

47

to come around when she gets ready to nurse. They are very strong minded and want to nurse all the time. The mama isn't ready and will ignore them. But when she's ready, she lays down and grunts in this special way as if to say, "OK, it's time now. Let's everybody have dinner." It's a wonder to behold. Then, when she gets through, she gets up and one or two of the piglets will still be hanging on, trying to get a little more. She just goes about eating her corn and doing her things, ignoring them. It is fascinating to watch. Once they are grown and reach a certain size, she ignores them. But even then, I can tell that she recognizes her own, well up until they are almost grown.

Horses, though not as smart as mules, are still pretty aware. I have noticed that horses like to greet each other. I had two horses, Dolly and Pet, mother and daughter, and they could be away from each other two years. When they met, it was like a reunion. "I'm so glad to see you." And how they would nuzzle each other. Of course, Pet had nursed until she was over two years old. After I had Pet broke and was riding her somewhere, if I took the bridle off and didn't watch, she would stand around nursing on Dolly. Dolly didn't seem to mind. Pet was her baby. It looked funny, but then when Dolly had another colt, that was the end of it. But she let Pet nurse until she was about two and a half years old. They usually will be weaned at about eight or nine months old. It was interesting to watch that and to watch the relationship of Dolly to Pet's colts. When a new baby came, Pet always wanted to see it. "Well, you've got a new baby."

From observing animals a long time, I find that there is a natural pecking order. If you watch them long enough, you'll see that they learn how to interact with one another and to get along in whatever environment they are placed in. Power is not always expressed in physical strength. For example, Dolly, my little Choctaw Indian pony, managed to be the boss of the whole lot of horses and mules. We fed many times in wagons. We had the wagons out and put feed for the animals in them, and she controlled the herd even though she was so much smaller. There were big mules and big horses a lot stronger than her, and they tried to control her, but she learned how to get around. She knew how to get in a lick where it would hurt the most, and they learned to respect her. A big horse would kick over her back, and she would kick him right in the stomach. That was the end of that. She was the boss. She was small, but she learned how to make them all behave.

I have also found that animals are possessive. If there is a specific stall that belong to them, they like to have it. They don't like to have some other animal in it. They like their own space.

I learned, too, how mothers protect their young. Even a gentle old cow that is never prone to fighting will protect her calf if she is threatened. If a dog or colt comes up, her mother instinct will take over. The cow will keep her baby hidden and fight anything that comes up. The same is true of a mare. She will get her colt under her neck and whirl and kick and fight any intruder. These mothers never take into consideration their own safety. They will fight like tigers to protect their babies. This is an admirable quality that you see in animals.

Even mother chickens are good role models. It's the saddest thing of all today that youngsters can't watch an old hen with her little chickens. She'll cluck and scratch and show them, "Here's a bug. Here's something good to eat. Here's something over here." And then a hawk can come along, and she will make a certain sound, and all those little chickens will run and get under her wings and hide.

Animals are our last connection with other life forms. A child who is kept from having a pet is a deprived child. If there is a way to have pets, they will teach children responsibility, let them express love, and help them discover the natural order, and that is a beautiful relationship. It's part of a beautiful relationship with life as a whole.

6
How to Keep Dogs and Cats Healthy

The purpose of nutrition should be to support an animal with nutrients in order for him or her to have the best quality of life under the circumstances in which he or she exists. The goal should be a healthy animal with a shiny coat and a good disposition. Nutrition is the foundation of our treatment. If we cannot get the animal properly nourished, we are limited in the physical changes we can make and the behavior we can influence.

Modern day pet foods that are saturated with preservatives, food dyes, sweeteners, salt, and pesticides make the goal of good nutrition all but impossible to obtain. Some of these foods have been found to contain lead, mercury, aluminum, and arsenic. It is virtually impossible to maintain a state of harmony and well-being in an animal that is eating these kinds of foods. Garbage is still garbage, even if it does have vitamins and minerals added to it and some tasty chemical to attract the animal and make it addictive.

Making Your Own Food

Remember, no one can make a pet food as good as you can in your own kitchen. Almost daily, people tell me that they are told not to let their pets have food from the table, that it isn't good for them. My answer to that is this: If the food on your plate is harmful for your pet to eat, maybe you should not eat it yourself.

The important thing is to use fresh ingredients for making the food. Fresh doesn't mean expensive. The diet can be very simple. You can use a simple rule of thumb for combining ingredients, and proportions can be varied according to your situation, availability, nutritional need, season, climate, and weather.

For animals, as well as for humans, variety is the key to staying on the diet. Of course, you should tailor the diet to your animal's particular needs, not just take it out of a book or mechanically apply a formula or recipe.

Fulton, my cat, will sometimes catch a bird, which I don't like for him to do. I have a little mockingbird that is resident here, and the cat hates him, and there is a constant battle going on. The bird will dive bomb Fulton all the time. Fulton got her baby last year and killed it, and she's never forgotten it. I try to feed Fulton something to calm him down and fix it so the birds can live here, too, because I like them. The other night, the mockingbird sang all night long. I love to listen to her.

When we are eating, Fulton always seems to want to eat what we are eating. He eats green beans, leafy green vegetables of different kinds, and okra. He loves cantaloupe. If you are eating melon, he has to have some. I also give him some good quality commercial cat food, but I am supplementing that with all kinds of fresh foods, including brown rice and squash. He also has the run of the place and catches mice.

Fulton also loves green beans. We just hand them to him when we are eating them. He sits there. He thinks that when we eat, he should eat. We are bad parents, I guess, but we let him eat with us. We just let him sit there on the floor and hand food to him. He eats most of it. It's amazing. Then sometimes Helen (my wife) will tell him, "You didn't eat the last piece I gave you. You've got to eat that first." He will look at it, then look at her as if to say, "You expect me to eat that?" She'll pick it up and hand it to him, and he will eat it.

51

By putting your own love and energy into the food, you strengthen the relationship with your pet. This, of course, is the key to macrobiotic cooking in general. No amount of store-bought food, however natural and of whatever quality, can give that kind of love. Food prepared fresh each day with love is special. It carries a special vibration, and the person or animal who eats it absorbs that energy.

Homemade food does not need preservatives. It can be made with the freshest ingredients, such as grain that has been freshly ground. You can get a small home grinder for this. In this way, feeding time becomes a special event. It is a time when you can express your love and be loved by your animal.

If it is not convenient to prepare food daily, several days' rations can be prepared in advance and placed in the refrigerator, though this will reduce its *ki*, or life energy. Add a little warm water and possibly some fresh leftovers from the table, and you have a warm meal.

You will reap enormous personal satisfaction by doing this for your pet. Even if you have to use a commercially prepared food because of lack of time or convenience, you can modify the diet by adding fresh ingredients and the same kind of foods that you and your family are eating every day. The effects on your pet's health will be impressive. For guidelines appropriate for pregnant and lactating cats and dogs, see Chapter Seven.

The Pet Industry

Every year, Americans spend over four billion dollars on pet food. This is five times as much as is spent on cancer research. It is nine times as much as has been spent by the American Heart Association in its more than thirty years of existence, and four times as much as we spend helping the hungry nations of the world. In fact, the pet food industry was the fastest growing industry in America between 1976 and 1982. It is the largest single item in the supermarket and generates more profit than any other type of goods. It occupies more space than fresh fruits and vegetables. If you don't believe me, measure this space sometime in your local supermarket. You will be amazed.

Although extremely profitable, the pet food industry is totally unregulated. It has to answer to no one, and companies will do anything they can to get your animal to eat their food. I hate the word addiction, but this is their objective—to get your animal addicted to their food, so that when you go to the market and buy something else the dog or cat will only want that food. And if you bring something else in and the cat doesn't want it, you'll say, "Well, I won't buy that food any more, because the cat won't even eat it."

The situation in Canada is somewhat better. The Canadian Veterinary Medical Association monitors pet food. There is no comparable regulatory body in the United States. Needless to say, the pet food industry traditionally uses the cheapest, poorest-quality ingredients—ingredients that humans won't eat and that can't be used in some other way. Take protein, for example. By poor-quality protein, I am talking about digestibility. Skin leather is protein, but who wants to eat it? Chicken legs are another example. Chicken feet have very little meat in them, and are of a very poor quality. On pet food labels, they calla them "chicken parts." They grind the chicken feet and put them into dog food. There is so much chicken on the market now, so that's what the dog food companies use for protein a lot. That causes the animal to have problems. Many people don't realize that even dry pet foods have animal products and by-products in them. Even though they may be shaped like little stars or granules, they have this material cooked in. In modern society, there is still a widespread assumption that high protein food is better, especially for pets, but this isn't so.

If you watch young golden retriever puppies, they seem to have what I call periodic lamenesses in their legs. That is an indication that they're not getting enough calcium, so you must increase the amount of seaweed in their diets. You have to watch for that, because if you don't, the body will pull calcium from the bones, creating problems. Aduki beans are a good source of calcium, as are lentils, chickpeas, and leafy greens. They can be used regularly. Down in this part of the country, we have a little red pea that's very strong. It is almost like an aduki bean and can be used occasionally. Bigger beans, such as lima beans and black-eyed peas, can be cooked for your pets occasionally, but not on a daily basis.

Additives

In addition to poor-quality ingredients, which are high in fat and cholesterol and low in vitamins, minerals, and other essential nutrients, most commercial pet foods contain additives and preservatives. These extend shelf life—and thus profits—but not the life or health of your pet. On the contrary, they reduce the life of the animal—and hence the health of the owner—by creating endless side effects and problems that turn up down the line. In fact, there are more additives and preservatives in pet foods than in any foods on the market. Just read the fine print on your typical cat food or dog food label. It reads like a chemical dictionary.

Let's look at a few examples. MSG—monosodium glutamate—is routinely added to many pet foods. The purpose of MSG is to enhance taste and make the food appear better than it is. The price for this is high. It induces the animals to eat more. It can cause some animals to lose weight. It can cause a sense of stomach fullness, belching, distension, numbness, general weakness, palpitations, cold sweats, and throbbing in the head. MSG can also lead to eye or brain damage, as well as to stunted skeletal growth, marked obesity, and female sterility.

Sodium nitrate and sodium nitrite are chemical preservatives and color fixatives. Sodium nitrate is less dangerous, but can easily convert to sodium nitrite, which is more toxic. Sodium nitrite is associated with decreased storage of vitamin A and carotene in the liver, permanent epileptic-like seizures, permanent reduction in brain activity, and severe arthritic pains, to name a few of its side effects. It also combines with hemoglobin to form methemoglobin and causes a lack of oxygen in the cells. Sodium nitrite is also linked with causing cancer throughout the body.

BHT—butylated hydroxytoluene—is another common preservative found in our commercial pet foods. It has been known to cause decreased growth rate, weight loss, brain damage, eye damage, liver damage, edema of the chest and breathing difficulties, and abnormal behavior patterns in puppies, if eaten by the female during pregnancy.

BHA—butalated hydroxyansole—contributes to weight loss, retards growth rate, and inhibits contraction of the smooth muscles of the intestines.

These are just a few of the chemicals in our nation's pet foods. After all of the medical and scientific tests showing their harmful effects, their continued presence on the market is a mystery to me. So long as we, the general public, buy them, there is excessive profit to be made. Making your own pet food or using more natural-quality pet food from a company you can trust will help reverse this appalling trend and immeasurably improve the health of our dogs, cats, and other pets.

Better-Quality Pet Food

Things are gradually getting better. I am encouraged that people are asking more about the quality of foods. Now they are asking more about the quality of their dog foods, too. Here is a good example. Recently I have noticed that people are comparing the different breeds of dogs and wondering whether they should all be fed the same thing. One company is beginning to make specialty foods, and one is promoting a special dog food for small dogs. We are going to become more specific than that and that's going to be good. People are willing to pay for good quality. It's when people are gypped or when they feel someone is trying to hoodwink them that they object.

Here is another encouraging sign. When I first suggested many years ago that we have Dr. Mark Morris down to speak to us on nutrition at a veterinarian's meeting, I was almost laughed out of the room. Back then I was concerned with diet.

That was over thirty-five years ago. I felt real bad, and I said to myself, "That's their problem." Eventually things change. I have been saying for twenty-five years that hip dysplasia has a nutritional base. Now you would be surprised how other veterinarians are gradually coming around. Pet food companies are beginning to say that their food is better because it helps prevent this sort of thing. They don't want to lose customers, so they are changing. Overall we are seeing a better picture. Natural pet foods may not become mainstream in my lifetime, but it will happen. It's going to happen and we are evolving in that direction, and I am really pleased to see it.

The people whose commercial pet food I was using went into bankruptcy and their quality went down. I could tell. That's the thing we have to watch in commercial foods, even the so-called natural ones. They get to where they need a little more profit. They cheat, and there is no regulation, nor am I sure we should have any. Regulations just encourage people to find ways around them. Still, there are a lot of pet food companies that use harmful chemicals. This is one of the things that a pet owner has to be aware of. I wonder especially about the quality of oils and fats in the so-called natural pet foods. I'm now getting a food product made in California called Nutrimax. It contains lamb and chicken, but it is a special chicken that has been raised free of all antibiotics and is free of all drugs. Still, I don't give much of it to an animal. I'll give a cat only about a teaspoonful.

Making the Transition to a Better Diet For Your Pet

As a rule, I try to make all transitions gradual so as not to shock the system. If I know the animal is eating a diet that is very toxic, I do not make a drastic change. Otherwise, you may precipitate a healing crisis. Sometimes I have to do that, but I also warn the owner, because if a healing crisis occurs, the animal will get sicker. Then you have a very unhappy owner who may do all kinds of crazy things. I try to make the transition gradually, especially with cats, because you can get the animal to refuse all food if you are not careful. I will usually ask owners to start adding some of the new diet into what they have been feeding them, gradually changing it over a period of about a week. Usually it will take that long. With a dog, it is much easier to do. You can usually have a dog eating something different in two or three days, but cats are more difficult, and sometimes it is almost impossible. They don't understand, and their taste buds have become accustomed to their current food.

We don't talk about it a lot, but there really is an addiction factor with animal foods. Recently, a drug salesman said to me, "Oh, doctor, you get their tastebuds trained like this, and they will be coming back and back and back." He didn't know that he was losing the sale right then, because I don't want to addict people's animals to any drug or chemical. This violates my basic integrity.

With the cat, I will start by adding a little brown rice into the diet. If the cat's never had brown rice, I'll just have them put in a tiny amount and see what happens. Some cats are easier than others. It's amazing to me how cats respond to the bringing in of new things—food, a new pet, a change in the household. I can usually trace these influences. This week I had a cat in that had a history of being a playful, wonderful individual and of playing very well with the family dog. But then the dog got bigger, and so the family felt they needed to get another dog as a companion for the first dog. Ever since they brought the new dog in, the cat has been belligerent and withdrawn. She has a fairly rough hair coat. She eats sporadically. So they decided to bring in another cat for her to play with. The cat that they brought in was an outgoing cat. The animal resents the new cat, fights him, and doesn't want him around her. He tries to play with her, but she doesn't respond.

My approach to this is to stimulate the digestive system with homeopathic remedies while introducing changes in the diet. Just this week, for the first time, this cat indicated that she might play with the other cat. She wasn't eating anything, though they kept all kinds of things out for her to eat. I took away all of the things that I thought were bad, including some heavily chemicalized food. Then I let her have some food that used to be one of her favorites while introducing new things in small portions, and now she likes that. She doesn't eat regularly yet, but at least she is eating. Her attitude is also beginning to change. The homeopathic remedy that I was using is helping her get over her anger and resentment. We are finding that she is going to accept this cat and wants to play with him. I have asked the owners to separate her food away from the other cat's—to remove it completely and offer this better quality food. Now she has indicated that she would like to play with him. She still has not been on the food long enough to develop a better hair coat, but she will in thirty days, if she continues to eat this way.

Over the years, I've found that people tend to go to extremes. Either they give their pet really bad food and say, "I don't have time," or they neglect the animal. They tell me, "I just couldn't feed it, so I had to wait twenty-four hours." That throws the animal off its feeding schedule. Then I have had people whose jobs change. I had one client who was very cooperative, but then suddenly her hours changed, and she didn't get home from work until early in the morning. We had to change the feeding schedule for the cat because of her working hours. This greatly affected the animal. She had been working during the day and in the evening she would come home and eat her own meal and sit before the TV. The cat would sit on the couch next to her and eat its meal. The woman and the cat ate at the same time. Suddenly this routine changed, and the cat became less healthy.

While normally it is a good idea to give your cat food that is prepared fresh every day, it is not always convenient, especially if you are working all week or are the only person in the house. I find that under these circumstances you can prepare some of the cat's food up to several days ahead of time if you have a good refrigerator. Prepare the grain and the animal protein and package them separately. I don't like freezing, but in one case I allowed someone to freeze the meat. He would take out a portion of the meat, thaw it, and feed it to his pet. That worked out fine. He found that it worked out better to keep the foods separate and then mix it up just before serving rather than store it all together.

I modify things quite a bit, depending on the owner, the home, and the work situation. I had one client who had ten or twelve cats, and I had her cooking for all of these animals. They were doing great, and then all of a sudden she didn't want to cook for them anymore. The cats didn't understand, and that created a big problem. She put them back on commercial cat food, and some of them got real sick. The change in diet shocked their systems.

I wracked my brain figuring out how to deal with this situation. I finally told the lady to take a teaspoon of the fresh food that was left and put in just that tiny amount with the commercial cat food. That helped reduce the shock to the cats. I had to make a compromise. It wasn't ideal, but it helped the cats adjust to the new situation.

In giving meat to a cat, I like for it to be ground up. This makes it easier to digest. Now I realize that in nature the animal takes meat off the bone, along with the hair. If a person has beef on the bone, it's all right to let the cat pull it off. They enjoy trying to handle it themselves. But generally people don't have beef like that these days. I advise them to take the meat, put it in water with a tiny bit of sea salt, and just boil it. The cats really seem to enjoy the beef broth, too.

When changing your cat's diet, the main thing is to be flexible and not meet the cat head on. If the cat says, "I'm not eating this," don't say, "If you don't eat that, you starve!" No; give in, I advise, because you can go around it. You can find something that the animal will eat. If their taste buds are set for something and you try to overpower them, you are wasting good time. I hope these general hints will be of some use to pet owners.

7
Prenatal Care and Birthing

The care of kittens and puppies should start with the diet of the mother even before conception. The prenatal life—life from conception to birth—is the most important time in the life span of the individual. It is in this stage that the constitution is formed. This constitutional influence is felt for the entire life of the organism.

The number of animals that we are seeing with nutritional problems is increasing at an alarming rate. Virtually no attention is being paid to prenatal nourishment of the fetus. In dogs and cats, there are only about two months to build a complete animal. The average gestation period for dogs and cats is from 58 to 63 days. If that mother has not been on a good, natural, nutritional diet, and is she has some deficiency carried over from her own mother, you can only expect harmful and often disastrous results, such as birth defects, weak constitutions and so on.

More attention should be given to prenatal nutrition. Postnatal nutrition is important, too, but the constitution is being formed in the prenatal state, and no matter how good the postnatal state, the influence of the prenatal state will, to some degree, shape the animal's entire life.

Recently a young doctor was asked why so many premature babies were being born today. He replied, "When the apple is ripe, it will fall." To me that statement reflected complete ignorance. The importance of nutrition cannot be overemphasized. The work of Dr. Weston Price is very important; he is a dentist who studied primitive diets and the dental arch in people and confirming that food is critical to the development of dental structure. He found that as humans began to live in a more industrialized society and eat more processed foods, the dental arch began to change, resulting in some of the jaw and teeth spacing problems seen today. Similar abnormalities are turning up with increased frequency in pets. Undershot and overshot jaws and retained baby teeth, along with juvenile vaginas, retained testicles, mental retardation, and hip dysplasia are seen daily in a large practice.

The lack of attention to prenatal nutrition is causing havoc in our pet community. The abnormalities listed above are just some of the evidence we see daily. Sometimes we are taught to look in the wrong places for the cause. For example, it is taught in modern veterinary medicine that an undescended testicle in the male animal is a sex-linked problem that is transmitted by the genes of the female. Granted, there may be some genetic influence, but the real problem is in the prenatal nutrition. If the mother already has a deficiency in her makeup, she has no choice but to transmit a part of that deficiency on to her young, regardless of her diet. But proper nutrition is a step in the right direction to correct a problem that may take several generations to reverse completely.

In over forty years of practice, I may have seen an undescended testicle in one cat. I attribute this to the ability of the cat to be a hunter, adding small insects and rodents to the diet and thus avoiding the pitfalls of the modern way of eating. However, with more confinement of the cat, along with the spraying of insecticides to kill insects, the cat is being denied this avenue of nourishment. The result is that we have seen more undescended testicles in the last year than we had seen in the previous forty years. The warning signs should be very plain.

Selecting a Pet

The importance of good parents that are healthy and vigorous cannot be overemphasized in selecting a pet or in getting your puppies or kittens off to a good start. Of course, much will depend on the breed. Things to consider and questions you should ask yourself include the following:

- Could this animal easily adapt to my living conditions?
- Where did the breed originate?
- Is the breed adaptable to this climate?
- What was the original purpose of the breed?
- Am I willing to make the sacrifices that would make the animal's life safe, healthy, and pleasant?
- Why am I drawn to this animal?
- Am I asking for trouble?

There are several classes of dogs. There is the sporting dog which hunts primarily by scent. There are the terriers and hounds. There are working dogs and non-working dogs. There are toys and miniatures. This is the reason it is foolish to talk about "dog food." It's important that we understand that there are all these types and backgrounds. When we change the natural purpose or setting of the animal, we have to take this into consideration. We constantly put animals in situations for which they were not originally bred or acclimated. Asking them to perform in such an environment puts them in a terribly stressful situation.

A perfect example is taking the St. Bernard and bringing him to Texas. He has a big, heavy coat, which was originally bred and suited for use in the Swiss Alps. You bring a St. Bernard to Texas and give him high-protein food, and it's like putting high-octane gasoline in a car that was not made for it and then racing the motor. The animal suffers terribly in hot, humid climates.

Now the Chihuahua, on the other hand, is native to Mexico and more acclimated to the heat. He takes it very well. I have actually seen a Chihuahua go into a coma after being left in an air-conditioned house. They don't tolerate cold very well. They need more concentrated food and they need more heat. These are extreme examples, but typical of our modern inappropriate behavior.

The other day someone asked me about keeping an Italian greyhound as an apartment dog. In this case, you are needlessly confining an animal that needs to run. Unless you have some way to take him or her out regularly to run, the dog will not adapt well to an apartment. You need a more docile animal, one more suited to the indoors, like a cocker spaniel. Even a beagle that's supposed to run rabbits can tolerate an apartment better than an Italian greyhound, because he runs, but not that much. It's hard on animals that are bred for running or herding to be put in a situation where they can't express their true natures.

In addition to that, feeding such an animal a diet that's high in protein (and thus creating the need for strong activity) puts a tremendous stress on that body. When you take a dog that is confined and feed it meat, toxins accumulate and stress develops. As my grandmother used to say, "If you want to make a dog mean, tie him up and feed him raw meat." What you are actually doing is making him more yang, and he wants to express himself. He wants to get out and move with all that energy. If you take the animal out, it is happier.

But the dog's whole system may still be under stress, depending upon what you are feeding him. Biologically, digestion in a sedentary animal is usually incomplete, and incompletely digested food becomes toxic. First, you will see it expressed in the teeth; then you will see it expressed in the other parts of the body—sometimes in the skin, sometimes in the soreness in the muscles, and so on. It is an incomplete digestion, much as you would have in a car that is not built for burning high-octane gas.

Over time, these toxins build up in the body, and they are not something that you ordinarily see. The pet owner thinks that everything is going along fine, and yet toxins are building up very rapidly and can cause trouble. First, it will be manifest in the teeth, usually in the form of an accumulation of plaque, and then discharge occurs, sometimes in the eye, sometimes in the skin. These are some of the areas you can watch for signs of toxicity. Someone sensitive to it can see it. By working with the diet, I've been able to adjust things like that for animals.

For example, if I feel an animal is suffering from too much protein and from protein that is poor quality, I will add something like tofu to the diet to cool him down. In addition to tofu, yin vegetables like cabbage, kale and leafy greens are another way to help him relax. Leafy vegetables that are cooked or lightly boiled or steamed work well.

Let's take a sporting or hunting dog, and assume you are trying to make a pet out of it. Give her this high-protein dog food and pen her up in a small area and you will soon have problems. Now if the dog could get out and run for half a day, she would burn off a lot of the drosses or toxins, and it wouldn't be nearly so hard on her. But if you don't have anything but a city park to walk him in two or three times a week or even everyday, you need to look at how much of that toxic condition you are creating in her. All of that high metabolic energy has to go somewhere, and when her body doesn't adjust, the next thing you know it will be expressed in her skin, tissue, or organs. A dog like that really needs to be outside every day, to chase things and play, to really work out. I have seen Irish Setters hunt all day long. It takes an animal that is especially bred to do that. The labrador retriever, the Weinereimer, and other pointers and setters should not be put in confined situations. In such circumstances, the best you can do is make the dog's diet more yin and try to adjust it so that he's not miserable. Even when these working breeds are under working conditions, they can have trouble metabolizing processed fats. Ninety-eight percent of their skin problems are traceable to poor fat metabolism. Processed fats and hydrogenated fats are a strange fare for the body.

In contrast, spaniels are more docile. They are smaller and can adjust better to less activity. It still doesn't mean that they don't need the exercise; they do, but they can adjust to a situation better than one of those dogs that is bred for all day hunting.

The Pregnant Cat

The animal will usually eat a larger volume of food. Ordinarily, I recommend feeding the adult cat fifty percent animal food, twenty-five percent grains, and twenty-five percent vegetables (see Chapter 9 for a more complete description of the adult diet). Include some seaweed to provide the trace minerals. One cat we really concentrated on had beautiful kittens. This indicated to me that getting the diet straightened out even before the animal is pregnant will keep deficiencies from developing, both in the mother and the offspring.

A variety of seaweeds, including Irish moss, kelp, and dulse, can be offered. This ensures that all essential nutrients are provided. For a long time I got seameal from Wachner's. The gentleman who started Wachner's was a concert pianist and was having a great career when he found out he had a terminal illness. He started investigating primitive diets and as a result developed this line of seaweed supplements.

Now there are other seaweeds that you can use; you don't have to have that particular source. It's expensive but I like nori for cats. They seem to love it; it smells like fish. Roast it a little bit, crumble it, and sprinkle it over their food or mix it in.

Some people are concerned about increasing the calcium in the diet for pregnant animals. The seaweed has a lot of calcium in it and it's organic calcium, which seems to be readily available to the body. The big problem we have with calcium is that there are inorganic and organic forms. Again, I think we need to go back and listen to nature. Nature puts organic minerals in the plant, and then the animal gets them from eating plants. We always have to remember the chain of events. We have to realize that the mineral kingdom supports the plant kingdom, and the plant kingdom supports the animal kingdom. If we start trying to skip one of the steps, we get into difficulty.

The same dietary recommendations hold true for the nursing cat. The only difference in the diet would be an increase in the volume of food. When I have an animal that I know is pregnant or is going to be pregnant, I usually put them on a powdered herbal mixture called Birth Aid which contains red raspberry leaves as the primary ingredient and a small amount of dried dandelion. This seems to strengthen the mother's body and gets her ready for delivery. It's something herbalists have known for centuries. I like to give it to the mother through the lactating period as well because the reproductive systems needs to adjust itself and return to normal following the birth experience. It seems to help prevent problems.

Of course, you can also mix your own herbs. Sometimes I take a two-finger pinch of the dried dandelion and put it into the food. You could also make a tea out of it, by taking a teaspoon of the powder and putting it in about a cup of water. Bring it to a boil and let it steep for a few minutes. Then add a teaspoon of that mixture to the food. But I find that, as long as I don't put in too much of the dried, powdered herbs, they just eat it and don't pay any attention to it. That's what I would rather do, just mix the powder in.

Cats are individualistic. What one will eat, another won't, and you have to understand that. If an animal seems to object to something, then I try to live with the objection and go around it rather than force them to eat it. You have to start from where you are, and then you can slowly change the diet. If an animal on a very poor diet becomes pregnant and you make a drastic change in their diet to one of better quality, they may begin to discharge toxins into the bloodstream, which will have a deleterious effect on the young. So it's much better to have them on a good diet before they become pregnant.

For an adult cat that is pregnant and on a commercial food diet, you can begin to add something natural and unprocessed. Examples would be a teaspoonful of grated raw or lightly steamed carrots, chopped-up leafy greens, or round vegetables like cabbage or squash. And then you could add twenty to twenty-five percent raw or lightly cooked fish. I prefer the white as opposed to the blue fish, and I try to stay away from tuna. It contains mercury and has a much stronger energy than white fish.

The Pregnant Dog

Usually a puppy should be weaned after six weeks. Through some feeding trials that we did here, we found that puppies and kittens ate early if they had adequate prenatal nutrition. In Western medicine, we have not had enough emphasis on prenatal nutrition—the environment and condition under which the mother exists. This is taught in Chinese medicine. If we get the mother in good condition, she is going to convey good immunity to the offspring. She's going to have good strong puppies, and those puppies can take a vaccine. If the nutrition of the mother is not right, then deficiencies will manifest in the young regardless of how good the nutrition is later on.

For an average sized-dog, like a golden retriever, I would start to check the mother even ninety days before she conceived. I'd examine her for any physical defects that would suggest nutritional deficiencies. For example, I'd check that her vulva is completely and nicely developed. I'd check her eyes and ears. Then I'd start her on a good diet. By a good diet, I mean that I would have her taking about fifty to sixty percent grains, and if she is a big dog, I could use some corn, some oats, some barley, and about twenty-five percent meat of good quality. Then I would have her taking about twenty-five percent freshly steamed, locally grown vegetables that were in season. In addition, because of the mineral deficiencies of our soil due to repeated cultivation, I would introduce some seaweed into her diet. I would also want her to have sesame oil or safflower oil, one of the better oils, as opposed to animal fats, because the body—whether human or animal—has problems with animal fat. The essential fatty acids in good-quality oils are very necessary.

Ideally, I'd maintain her on this diet for sixty to ninety days before breeding. During her gestation period, I would be guided by the amount of food she craves. Let her more or less tell you how much to feed her. Then after she is pregnant, I would introduce red raspberry leaves as a supplement, because a small amount of raspberry leaves seems to strengthen the reproductive system. You can get these in a powdered form. As mentioned in the preceding section on pregnant cats, you can use this as a tea or a powder. This will strengthen the reproductive system and make birthing of the young easier.

False Pregnancy

False pregnancy, or psuedocyesis, is a condition where the animal has all the appearances of being pregnant but isn't. It is seen more often in dogs than in cats. However, it does occur in cats. It usually occurs about thirty to sixty days following a heat period. The breasts develop, the disposition will usually be crabby, and the abdomen enlarges. The average owner naturally expects that his animal is pregnant and will give birth to kittens or puppies. However, it doesn't occur.

If you suspect that your pet has this condition, I suggest you take it to your veterinarian for an examination. Sometimes we have only a matter of hours in which to do surgery and remove the uterus to save the animal's life.

However, if your animal is a valuable breeding animal, or if you want it to have young in the future, you can use a combination of an herbal cleansing formula and a poultice and a ginger compress. It consists of equal parts of the following herbs: Cascara sagrada, echinacea, slippery elm bark, and cayenne, and ginger (all in powder form). Combine all the ingredients and sift together three times. Then fill number-two-sized capsules by placing the powder mixture in a shallow bowl, taking one half of a capsule, placing the open end in powder, and pressing against the bottom of the bowl until that part of the capsule is full. Then take the other end of the capsule and tip into the powder to get a small amount to fill the end of that half. Then put the two pieces together. The capsule should be packed full and fit tightly. Give one capsule of this herb combination twice daily for a cat or a small toy breed dog. Larger dogs would get proportionately more.

The ginger compress should be applied as hot as the animal can stand it, in an area just below the navel and back to the flank. This should be applied for at least ten minutes. Follow the ginger compress with a taro potato plaster over the same area. Leave the taro plaster on overnight, if possible. I usually apply this under an orthopedic stockinette, but an old sock or sweater will do to hold the plaster in place.

A vaginal discharge may occur. Consider this a good

symptom and continue the treatments daily. Twice a day is even better. After the discharge has stopped and the animal has lost some weight, we are ready to put the animal on a prenatal diet to get her ready for mating. Always keep in mind that this is a dangerous situation, and you may have to give the animal surgery to save her life. This program is an alternative to surgery, if there is sufficient time and the situation is not critical. When progress is not being made, I suggest surgery and complete removal of the uterus and ovaries. This can be a real disappointment if you were planning to raise kittens or puppies. If you have a cat, you can take heart, because this condition is rare in cats. I've seen it in cats only about two or three times in thirty-five years. But it is quite common in dogs. This could be due to the cat's ability to be a hunter, by which she can modify her diet some, and also due to the ability of the cat to exercise her body by stretching. This helps burn off some of the toxins that accumulate in the more sedate dog. Also the cat is less likely to eat "junk," whereas the dog is a scavenger. Commercial pet food doesn't help, and may be a contributing factor to false pregnancy in both dogs and cats. So this is another reason to make your own pet food using the freshest, most natural ingredients.

When you choose a pet, look for signs of good health. Evidence that an animal's mother had good prenatal nutritional care includes early development, a high degree of intelligence, and a calm mental attitude. Once the selection of an animal has been made—type, breed, age, sex, etcetera—make changes in its diet gradually. Concentrate on the animal's strong points. The younger he or she is, the easier it is to correct weaknesses. Always reflect on whether you are doing the best by your animal—and yourself. A good question to ask yourself is, Why am I drawn to this animal? Look in the mirror. Have someone make a picture of you and your new puppy or kitten and study the picture. You may be surprised at what you discover.

8
Kitten and Puppy Care

Growing up on the farm, I can't recall that we ever had a sick cat or dog. My grandmother's cats and dogs were healthy hunters. Most just died of old age. One dog my grandmother had given a man was shot because it had developed "running fits." My grandmother commented, "That dog got sick just like that man got sick, from eating that old white flour. I won't make that mistake again." She refused when he wanted another puppy.

The birth of young on the farm was always an exciting time for me, whether it was a litter of kittens in the hay barn, an old sow with a brood of pigs in the woods, or a new baby colt in the pasture. Each one had to have a name. Usually my sisters and I had them named by the very first day.

We need to keep certain basics in mind when we take care of kittens and puppies. The main tenet is that the mineral kingdom supports the plant kingdom, and the plant kingdom supports the animal kingdom. Therefore, if we have sick soil, we will invariably have sick animals. The conclusion is clear: if we can do so, we should raise our own food organically, both for ourselves and our pets. If we do not have such an opportunity, the next best thing is to seek foods from sources grown without pesticides and chemicals.

Generally, kittens and puppies will open their eyes between nine and fourteen days. Once we took a mother cat that had one litter of kittens and was from all outward appearances a normal, healthy individual. We put this mother cat on an excellent diet. None of the ingredients contained any chemicals or insecticides. We combined the ingredients in the diet in the approximate proportions by measure. Good quality meat came to about fifty to sixty percent, and steamed fresh vegetables twenty-five percent. The mother cat was especially fond of grated cooked carrots and also ate some cooked onions, broccoli, cabbage, and cauliflower. The last twenty-five percent of her diet was cooked brown rice, and occasionally she was given some barley soup, poured over the rice and mixed in with the other ingredients. To this we added some seaweed powder. Approximately one-eighth teaspoon of powdered seaweed was given in one feeding daily.

The results shocked me! The kittens began opening their eyes the second day. They were active, but calm and quiet. The seventh postnatal day, they demanded and ate solid food. The litter seemed to do everything early. They weaned themselves at about five weeks. I followed the litter as long as I could. I have now lost contact with all but one of the litter of five. All of these kittens were exceptional. Everybody who saw them would make some comment on their beauty and intelligence. It has now been seven years since we completed these feeding trials. The one cat we still follow is considered by her owners to be a "super cat."

On the farm, my grandmother always gave her cats the milk from any cow that was a new freshener. That is to say, she gave them the milk from any cow with a newborn calf. She usually did this for about nine days following the birth of a calf. She also used this new milk for any weak or sick animal she was trying to nurse back to health. Now I know that this milk was rich in vitamins, minerals, and antibodies from the cow and is called colostrum. She could perform miracles with "new milk," as she called it.

It should go without saying that the first food for any young animal should be its mother's milk. I recall that once my father bought a small jackass to raise for a breeding animal. They bred mares to jackasses in those days to raise a crossbreed called a mule for pulling plows in farming and pulling wagons for transportation. At any rate, this was a very young jack. He was only about four months old when Dad brought him home. He wouldn't or couldn't eat the corn that was offered him, and he wasn't doing well at all. My father was concerned that he might lose the animal.

I recall the moment exactly when my grandmother said. "That jackass needs some first milk." She had a cow freshen in a day or two, and she proceeded to teach that jack ass to drink cow's milk. He made a rapid recovery, and even after he was grown, he would bray when he heard the rattle of milk buckets in the milk barn.

Nursing

The very first food that the kittens, or any other young animal, must take is milk from the mother's breast. This milk contains a very high concentration of vitamins, minerals, and antibodies produced by the mother. The healthy kitten will have the natural instinct to nurse the mother, and if left alone with her will find its way to the breast. I never cease to be amazed at the strength of this first milk.

The same thing goes for puppies. All baby animals need the first milk from their own mother. The first milk from another species is helpful if the animal's own mother is not capable of nursing. The concentrated vitamins will be there, but the antibodies the animal so desperately needs at this time will not transfer to another species. The ideal thing to do would be to secure a substitute mother of the same species. The first milk or colostrum is present in the milk only the first few days following birth. Thus, even if the substitute mother is of the same species, if her young were born more than ten days to two weeks earlier, her milk will not contain the protective colostrum that it did immediately following birth.

The reflex to nurse the mother, the suck reflex, is present in all healthy newborns. If the reflex to nurse the mother is not present in the baby, it means something is constitutionally wrong. If the newborn fails to nurse for any extended period of time, it seems to lose the suck reflex or at least it seems to diminish. I have seen the suck reflex reestablished, but it is difficult. A few drops of mother's milk will sometimes do wonders.

72

The constitution of an animal can be defined as the qualities the animal was born with. These are largely determined in the womb. The condition of an animal can be defined as those qualities acquired after birth. It could be a healthy condition due to a strong constitution, or it could be a sickly condition due to a weak constitution. Animals with weak constitutions seem to invite invasive organisms. Those with strong constitutions tend to have healthy conditions, and even though they are subjected to extreme conditions only tend to get stronger and survive. Puppies and kittens exposed to extreme conditions early in life who successfully adapt to these circumstances appear to take conditions in stride during their entire lives. The husky, the Malamute, the leopard hound, and some of the hunting hounds are good examples of animals with this strong capacity for survival.

In looking for signs of a weakened constitution, the first thing to be aware of is that a fat puppy is not necessarily one with a strong constitution. Fat is not even a good indication of the animal's condition. Mental alertness, bright eyes, and interest in the surroundings are the first qualities I would look for. The gait or walk is the next thing to be considered. Slow walking, abnormal gait, rabbit-hopping (where both back feet are brought forward at the same time), and other abnormalities are good indications of problems. Watch the hips and see if they seem loose and clumsy. Look in the mouth of the kitten or puppy and see if the palate seems higher than normal. Compare it with others. A high palate could be an early sign of a lack of mental and emotional development. Other signs that give us an indication later are undescended testicles or a juvenile vagina. These cannot be easily distinguished early, but over time are very important signs of nutritional deficiencies.

First Solid Food

The cat in nature was a hunter. It hunted for its food much as members of the cat family do today in the wild. The mother (or queen, as they are called) sought food by hunting small rodents and birds. After the kittens were about old enough to wean (between six and ten weeks of age), the mother cat would bring home a freshly killed bird or rodent and share it with her litter. The taste of fresh blood seems to stimulate young kittens. They then eagerly join the hunt for more food. They begin by catching small bugs and will pounce on almost anything that moves.

The mother dog in nature (or bitch, as she is called) would hunt and scavenge food. When she returned home to her litter, she would vomit up part of the food she had eaten. The pups would eat this upchucked food, and in this way were introduced to solid food. We see vestiges of this natural phenomenon at times in our domesticated dogs. Sometimes a mother dog will start vomiting up her food when her pups are about six to ten weeks old. If the mother is normal in all other respects and continues to eat, there is nothing to get excited about. If we then start feeding the puppies, the mother will compete with her own pups for food.

The male dog ceases to have an interest in the female after the heat and breeding period. He will compete for food but seems less aggressive during the mother dog's time of nursing the young. The mother dog in nature sought food from any source she could find. She would eat dead and decaying animals as well as small live animals, such as rabbits, squirrels, and other rodents.

Understanding nature can help us introduce solid food to our animals that have now evolved into human pets. Dr. Michael Fox has done some very good studies on dogs by studying wolves in natural settings. He has written several books which I highly recommend. I consider him one of the great minds in the veterinary health-care field today.

A good way of introducing solid food to young kittens is to take a small amount of ground beef, about the size of a small bean. Flatten this small bit of beef between the forefinger and the thumb and then dip the small bit of beef in egg yolk that you have previously separated from the white and placed in a small saucer. This egg-yolk-dipped beef bit is then placed in the mouth of each kitten. It is amazing how this seems to stimulate the animal's appetite for solid food.

Once solid food is introduced, kittens soon begin to lose interest in nursing. If adequate food is then provided, normal development takes place. The mother cat naturally begins to wean her kittens at about six weeks of age. On the other hand, if there is inadequate food, the mother tends to nurse the kittens longer. I have seen kittens from three successive litters still nursing the mother. I consider this abnormal and due to either an inadequate amount of food or some other dietary deficiency.

The introduction of solid food for puppies can also be accomplished by taking a small amount of ground meat, about the size of a pea dipped in egg yolk, and placing it in the mouth. This seems to stimulate the appetite of the average puppy. However, we should give some consideration to the animal's size, breed, origin, and purpose. For example, if I were dealing with a litter of Chihuahua puppies, I would prefer some ground chicken meat dipped in egg yolk instead of beef. If I were dealing with a litter of St. Bernards, I would use a larger portion of ground beef and possibly add a little cottage cheese before dipping the meat into the egg yolk. If the puppies were from one of the hunting or working breeds, my approach would be a bit different. If I were dealing with a litter of one of the bird-hunting breeds, I would introduce birds into the life of the puppies to carry over the ancestral memory of bird hunting.

If I were dealing with a litter of German shepherds, I would introduce solid food by using the small amount of raw ground beef that I described, and then would see to it that some raw meat was in their diet daily when they started eating solid food. I would continue this through adult life. I would start with the small portion, graduate to a level teaspoon, and then finally give a tablespoon daily in the adult diet, along with some lightly cooked, locally grown vegetables fed in the season in which they were grown. For example, root vegetables would be given more in fall and winter, and leafy vegetables more in spring and summer.

I like to feed kittens four times a day when they start taking solid foods. Frequent feeding helps to prevent overextension of the abdomen. By the time kittens are three to four months of age, the feeding times can be cut to two times a day. My personal preference is to feed a cat its main meal in late evening or early morning. The reason for this is that the cat was basically a night hunter, so it seems like a more natural time for feeding.

The feeding times for a cat can safely be cut to once a day at six to twelve months of age, though they often like to eat small amounts more often. It is a good idea to cut the other meals down in amount at first and then replace them with a tidbit when they are cut completely. I see no real harm in giving cats or dogs a small crunchy tidbit, so long as they do not contain preservatives or insecticides.

The dog's main food is generally best served in the afternoon. This is because the dog was basically a day hunter and scavenger. I abhor automatic feeders in which food is poured into a receptacle once a week and the animal is left to eat at will. I feel that feeding an animal should be an event. It helps to build an emotional tie and strengthen the human-animal bond.

Other Considerations

The importance of early human contact cannot be overemphasized. If you have the opportunity, I suggest that you start before birth by stroking the abdomen of the expectant mother and talking to the kittens in embryo. Soon after birth, stroking and massaging seems to have a mutual benefit in the human-animal bond.

The same can be said for puppies that are to become pets. The early socialization of puppies and kittens, as Dr. Fox and others have demonstrated, is very important. Isolation has detrimental effects. Both puppies and kittens learn in the first few weeks of life that there is a social order to things.

If you start with the pregnant mother, stroking her abdomen and saying loving words to her, there is little doubt in my mind that the unborn pick up the vibrations and develop a close tie with you after birth. On the other hand, if the mother is in a constant state of fear, it is very hard to overcome it in her young. This is why it is better to pick a kitten or a puppy from a family-raised litter than one from the puppy or kitten mills or even an adoption center. The adoption centers are necessary, and you do the animal a lifesaving favor in adopting it. Just be aware of the responsibility you are taking on, and give the animal an extra measure of patience and love. Be aware, too, that if the animal is a little older, you may never completely overcome some of the traumas that have been inflicted on it.

The importance of early human contact cannot be overemphasized. It can be mutually beneficial if the animal is handled in a loving, caring way. By stroking and loving a healthy pet, there is an interchange of energy that is of benefit to both the person and the animal.

Massage

My method of massage starts with gentle massage of the ears in a circular, clockwise fashion. There are two reasons for this. First, there is an acupoint in the ear for every major organ in the body. Therefore, as you gently massage the ears, you are in a sense stimulating or treating every major organ in the body. You are sending a minute electrical impulse (*ki*) to each organ. Second, the thermostat of the body is located near the base of the ear (triple heater points 16 and 17). By massaging the ear, we increase the *ki*, or energy flow, as well as the temperature of the body. You can experience this by rubbing your own ears.

Each ear represents one half of the whole body as well as the kidneys. We learn in acupuncture and macrobiotics that the kidneys control hearing. We also learn that the kidneys function best when warm. Therefore, it makes sense to warm the ears.

Once you have the energy up by massaging the ears, you may next gently stroke the animal from head to tail to direct the energy flow. You can do this daily for a house pet. Often when a problem is developing, a sensitiveness will appear in an associated acupoint or meridian, sometimes twenty-four hours before symptoms develop. By understanding this and being aware that your pet has suddenly developed a sensitivity to a given point, you can, through gentle massage, cause the energy to flow to the part and stimulate healing before a major problem develops.

Diet for Puppies

When the puppies are ten days to two weeks old, you can begin to introduce solid food. For a medium-sized dog like a golden retriever, I like to use about fifty percent grain and twenty-five percent good quality meat products. The animal is carnivorous, so I like that meat to be either barely cooked or raw. There was a great veterinarian who taught me this years ago down in Florida. As I said above, it's a good idea to take a little raw ground meat, dip it in the yellow of an egg, and put that in the dog's mouth. The dog will smack a time or two and soon begin demanding it. I'm not suggesting that you feed dogs just that, but it will stimulate their digestive system to develop and, before you know it, they will be wanting to eat solid food.

I start with that, and then I give fifty percent whole grain, twenty-five percent meat, and about twenty-five percent steamed, fresh vegetables. As I noted earlier, I like to use vegetables that are in season. For example, in winter I will use more root vegetables, like carrots, parsnips, and cabbage. Then in the spring, when the saps begin to rise, I will use more leafy vegetables and continue this on into the summer. As the seasons change, the diet can be adjusted accordingly.

Now, because we have cultivated our soils, there's always the possibility of mineral deficiencies. For that reason, I like to add the seaweed. I use that to provide the trace minerals and calcium that we're all concerned about.

If the puppy's small, it should be fed three or four times a day. Then, by the time it's six months old, you should be able to reduce its feedings to twice a day. And then by one year old, cut back to once a day and feed primarily in the afternoon if it's convenient. Again, we have to realize that the owner's work and hours vary, but a routine procedure where the animal is fed in the afternoon, and then let outdoors seems to work well. It can exercise and eliminate while outdoors, and this makes them more comfortable.

For puppies you can use any of the grains. Again, we go with the seasons. If it's winter (and very cold), we would probably add a little buckwheat because that helps produce heat in the body. We will use rice as the basic grain, but sometimes the owner can't afford it. In that case, you can use barley, whole oats, and even some millet, or you can use these grains in addition to rice from time to time. I find that these grains are very important, and if they are good quality, they make the basis for a very good diet. They create a very healthy animal and one that is brilliant. Rice always forms the basis. Corn gruel can also be used. When I was investigating this, I would go up and get the corn ground. It would still be warm from grinding. I was preparing the food in the kennel to feed the dogs, and I would love to use the freshly ground cornmeal.

The meat should be rare, but the grain should be cooked. It needs to be cooked to make it more digestible. I normally boil it. You can use a pressure cooker, and this would add more energy to it, which would be of value, too. Then once the grain is cooked, I add the vegetables and meat in just before feeding the puppy.

You can also feed the puppy leftovers. If you are eating a good diet, it's very good for the animal to act as a clean-up guy and share your food. It builds a very close bond between the person and the animal. Among the foods animals love most are aduki beans and aduki bean juice. It just seems to be magic. You don't need a lot, but it sure does help. This is very strong and a good source of protein. All of the foods that are prepared macrobiotically are excellent. The animal sees you eating this and often it will want some, too. Just mix it in, keeping to the proportions that I mentioned, because it maintains balance.

The oil the dog needs will be supplied naturally in this way. Fatty acids are required by the body. But there is an excess of animal fats in most dog food, and the animal's body has trouble handling them. The vegetable quality oils, such as sesame oil, corn oil, and natural oils in the grain and beans, will bring out the coat and are very good for the animal. We get into problems trying to get the body to accept fat from beef and pork and other animal quality foods. For a golden retriever-sized puppy, a teaspoonful of sesame oil daily in his diet is sufficient. The body can easily handle that quantity. This is much better than a processed fat of animal origin or than chicken fat, which the body will have trouble digesting, possibly resulting in skin problems, itching, and scratching. Finally, I would introduce a little seaweed, because even the best of our soils are deficient now. Seaweed provides trace minerals that might be missing from the food.

Special Foods

Brown Rice

As I've said, I like to use brown rice whenever possible. The protein that's in brown rice is very high quality, highly digestible, and moderate in volume. Because the animal is getting that high-quality protein, it doesn't require so much food.

If you are going to feed an animal brown rice, you should cook it and then blend it or run it through a food processor. Animals can't chew as we advise humans to chew in macrobiotics. You may chew your rice fifty times or more, but dogs and cats have the tendency to gulp food down. Blending it or putting it through a food processor will help them digest it much better.

Wheat Grass

Cats rarely have stomach problems, but they do have problems with proper elimination. Usually this is from a lack of fiber and of greens and vegetables in general. I have one client in New York who lives on the twelfth story of an apartment building with her and the cat doesn't get out. I have her raising wheat grass in the window, and that cat eats it; this gives her some fiber for her digestive system. My client says the cat is much better since she started that. "I don't try to make her eat it," she told me. "I just put it there in the window, and if she wants some, she eats it." If a cat has an opportunity to get out, it will eat grass and other greens that grow in the wild. But we have so much spraying now that you have to be careful, even if you have a nice lawn or park for your animal to run in.

Corn

Corn is, in some ways, more yin than wheat. But it also has its yang elements, and it has a lot of heat in it. If you are using corn, just realize that it does have that yang capacity, and then use something else such as leafy vegetables to balance and cool it down. this works very nicely to cool the animal down. When I was doing my feeding trials, I used a lot of cabbage and corn. They were available and inexpensive, and availability and cost have a lot to do with what we feed animals. The corn was plentiful, and I could have it ground. Then I cooked that. I got a lot of cabbage free from the vegetable market. It was nice, clean cabbage. They throw away the heart and the outer leaves, and in my opinion, those are the two best parts.

Kitty Litter and Training the Cat

Cats as a rule are very easily trained to a litter box. This training is usually easy, because of the natural tendency of cats to cover up their wastes. The box should be cleaned daily and the feces flushed down the toilet. If the litter box is not kept clean, the cat may decide to use some other part of the house for his toilet. Once this is done, it is very difficult to train the animal back to the litter box. If this should happen, I suggest that you first clean the area very well, and then apply one of the nontoxic pet repellents on the market, and add some valerian root tea to the litter box.

There are adaptation kits on the market for training cats to use the commode. Some people have been successful in using them.

There are many brands of kitty litter in stores today. I don't know that one is better than the other. However, you can use plain soil in the litter box. It's best to use sand if it is available. The commercial litter is usually inexpensive and often preferable to soil or sand because of its absorbent quality, but you want to be careful of harmful chemicals. The choice is yours. Good care of the litter box helps to control parasites.

If your cat is a male, you must make a choice concerning neutering. If you don't have the male cat neutered, you should know that he will begin to spray urine and to mark his territory at about six months of age. It is important to remember than if you wait until the male cat begins to spray and mark the territory, it is very difficult to train him away from urinating where he marked before, because of the urine odor. This can be true even if you have him neutered. My suggestion is to have him neutered before he begins to fight and spray.

Females, as a rule, are very easy to train to the litter box. They will, however, sometimes start using other areas to urinate. This is especially true if a female cat goes into heat and in so doing attracts a male, and if the male in turn marks his territory with urine. The female may then start urinating where the male has sprayed. Again, if this should happen, it is difficult to train her back to the litter box. I would use the valerian root tea to try to do this. It does no good to thrash or scare the animal with a newspaper or other weapon, and besides, it's cruel.

Dog Waste

Puppies should begin their training early. Six to seven weeks is a good time. Remember, you can control his bowels to some degree with feeding times. The natural thing is to have the urge to go immediately after eating. If you keep this in mind and immediately place him on the paper you are using to train him, things will go a lot more smoothly. If the dog is to use the yard, you should put him or her out immediately after feeding.

Feeding time should be training time. A few minutes devoted to this time will pay off handsomely down the line. If the animal is allowed to use the yard for his toilet duties, you should purchase a small tool for picking up the droppings and attend to this chore daily. The droppings can then be flushed down the toilet or, if you prefer, there is a small sanitary toilet that you can purchase and bury in the yard for the sanitary disposal of pet waste. If you use a public park for exercising your dog, be sure to take your poop scoop and a plastic bag along for collecting your dog's waste. Please do this, out of respect for others as well as for sanitary and health reasons. Nothing is more disgusting than stepping in animal waste when you are trying to enjoy a beautiful park. New York City was forced to pass an ordinance to require people to clean up after the pets they were walking in Central Park.

Responsible pet ownership includes looking after the animal's waste. Your pet should not be allowed to roam the property of others, either. If we do not respect the rights of others, we will face more and more restrictive laws. Respecting the rights of others is just as important as caring for and loving your pet.

Leash laws are on the books in most cities. They should be obeyed. We very often see animals seriously injured by another animal, a car, or an accidental shooting. The common excuse is, "I only let him out for a few minutes." I never say, but would like to, "If you had been looking after this animal properly, this would have never happened."

9

Determining What the Adult Animal Should Eat

I learned about feeding farm animals as a child. The fall was a great time on the farm where I grew up. As soon as the last of the crops were in, the gates were flung open, and all the animals were set free to go wherever they pleased. I noticed that the cows tended to head for the cotton fields, the horses for the corn fields, and the hogs for the peanut and sweet potato patch.

My grandmother explained to me that the cow had a compound stomach of four compartments, capable of digesting cotton stalks and leaves and even cotton and cottonseed. Horses, she explained, had a more simple digestive system, and even though they could digest grass fairly well, they could handle grain better. She explained that cows could handle more bulk, used their mouths to gather the bulk, and stored this food in one of the compartments of their stomachs. Later when they were lying down and resting, they belched up this stored food and chewed it well in the form of cud, and then reswallowed it for digestion. She even taught me to steal a cud from a healthy cow as she chewed it and to give it to one that was sick or not feeling well, or who had "lost her cud." She had me slip up to a cow lying down, grab her by the nose, thrust my hand into her mouth, and take her cud. She explained that it was safe to do this, as a cow has no upper front teeth—only a dental pad against which she collects grass and other rough material. A horse, on the other hand, has strong upper and lower front teeth that are capable of biting you severely.

Sheep and goats have pretty much the same tooth pattern as cows. Hogs have a strong snout for rooting and searching for food. I was amazed to observe an old sow eating hickory nuts, cracking them with her jaw teeth, separating out the goodies from the hulls, and never swallowing any of the hulls. I had trouble cracking those things with a hammer and picking them out with two hands and a pick.

I learned, then, to consider the teeth in determining an animal's diet. The tooth formula of the cat and dog is somewhat similar to those of farm animals. The teeth of the cat are smaller, as a rule, and sharper. This would indicate that the animal should have more meat in its diet. If we use the criteria of tooth size, shape, and purpose along with general body size, we should be able to figure out what an animal's diet should be from a natural point of view. We should be able to do this regardless of the animal's size, species, or place of origin. Even as a boy collecting animal skulls in the woods, I could pretty well figure out what the animals ate from the tooth patterns.

The way we did this was to use a formula, taking the total number of teeth as one hundred percent and then the number of teeth for each purpose as a percentage. For example, if the total number of teeth was thirty-two, four teeth were for tearing, four teeth for biting, and sixteen for grinding. This would be expressed as follows:

22 = 100% (total number of teeth)
4 for tearing = 25 percent (meat or foods to be torn
    apart before grinding)
4 for biting = 25 percent (softer foods such as fruit and
    vegetables)
16 for grinding = 50 percent (grains, nuts, seeds, and
    possibly crushed small bones)

Generally, there are three types of digestive systems found in nature. They are the simple stomach types we find in dogs and cats, the compound as we find in cows and related species, and the semi-compound we find in the horse, which allows him or her to handle grain and roughage; a large caecum is also present, which helps in the digestion of grass. Along with the teeth, the stomach type also helps determine an animal's diet.

If we take the total view, we can see that humans, too, are part of a biological system, one that is everchanging. Night changes into day, and day changes into night. Winter changes into summer, and summer changes into winter. In the Far East, this is referred to as changing from yin to yang and back to yin again. Therefore, the only constant we can depend on is change.

The biological system of which we are a part of is always seeking balance, trying to make adjustments for excess yin or excess yang. There is no static balance. Walter Russell observed this phenomenon and referred to it as the rhythmic balance interchange in nature. The Orientals simply say that the system is becoming more yin or more yang."

We can conclude that we live in a world of cause and effect. For every action, there is an equal and opposite reaction. If this is true, we can foresee or predict the results of an action, or trace it back to a cause. We can rest assured that violating the order of nature will eventually bring a compensation. We experience this in the form of sickness, an accident, or other unwanted change. Instead of looking at this as natural rebalance, we regard it as punishment.

It is my view that the increasing decline in natural immunity in animals and in humans is due to the widespread use of antibiotics, cortisone, and other medications and processed food. The virus that "invades" and "attacks" the immune system is a guest that we have unconsciously invited into our bodies through our lifestyle and diet.

The feeding of food unsuited for an animal's digestive system is a crime against nature, although that is a general statement and should not be taken too literally. Under certain circumstances, animals and humans have been forced to eat unnatural food, and their systems have evolved to allow the food to be readily accepted and utilized. A good example might be the Icelandic ponies that eat dried fish heartily, digest it, and have adapted very well to this unusual diet.

On the other hand, we know that feeding things to animals that they could not possibly get under natural circumstances creates problems. Not so long ago, I was visiting an East Texas ranch and saw the rancher feeding his cows liquid blackstrap molasses in a trough. Horse feed has been created that is sweetened with molasses. Dairy cows are fed high protein to make them give more milk. Where could a horse get syrup mixed with grain under natural conditions? Where could a cow get high-protein feed?

Feeding animals these unnatural foods causes some of the following conditions:

1. Creates attraction of mosquitoes and other parasites to the animal.
2. Causes stress on the body and, eventually, chronic deterioration of the natural immune system.
3. Antibiotics in particular kill off some of the bacteria in the animal's body. This causes a gain in weight, but at the same time the surviving harmful bacteria become very strong and turn into super bacteria. If the animal is consumed by another animal or person recently given antibiotics for some illness, a very dangerous situation can develop.
4. Processed sterile foods fail to feed the normal healthy bacteria in the bowel. If we further complicate the matter by residual antibiotics, either added to the food or just present in the product being fed, the normal bacteria flora in the bowel may be disturbed, weakening the digestive capacities of the animal.
5. Dr. John Ott has demonstrated the detrimental effects of artificial lights on plants and animals (such as fluorescent light) and the benefits of natural, full-spectrum light (such as sunlight). Pets kept in the house away from the sun may have problems in hair coat, general health, and reproduction.
6. The widespread use of chemicalized fertilizers, pesticides, and overcultivation has not only bankrupted the

American farmer, but also resulted in weaker farm products. Today it takes approximately 150 bushels of corn to equal the total digestible nutrients of just 100 bushels of corn at the end of World War II.

From a larger, more comprehensive view, we are part of a larger biological system that extends from the stars to the tiniest virus. This system, spanning the macrocosm and microcosm, is capable of correcting itself. This is the hope we have. For example, the lowly earthworm is capable of adding eighteen to thirty tons of nutrients per acre to the soil. This creature is capable of removing DDT from the soil as he adds valuable casts. Trees help clean the air by removing carbon dioxide and adding oxygen. Life itself is not a battle, unless we believe it is and create that kind of stressful warlike environment in our homes and communities.

Our pets are probably the most victimized creatures of all, because it is easy to play on our emotions. We are urged to protect them from fleas with flea collars around their necks that vaporize a deadly chemical, constantly stressing the liver and we give them pills for this or that "protection."The result is confusion in the public mind and sick and frightened animals.

How can I protect my dog or cat from fleas? How can I protect my pet from some dreaded disease? These are questions we hear daily. The truth is that an animal in a good state of health will have a natural resistance. If you see a problem developing, it is a good time to ask yourself, "Am I providing the essentials for a healthy animal?" These essentials are:

1. Clean, fresh water
2. Plenty of sunshine and fresh air
3. Wholesome, natural food
4. Moderate exercise

The following guidelines provide the foundation of a healthy diet:

Standard Guidelines

	Vegetables	Cereals	Animal Products
Adult Dog	25%	50%	25%
Adult Cat	25%	25%	50%
Geriatric	more	more	more
Growing	less	less	more
Yin Diseases	less	less	more
Yang Diseases	more	more	less
Hot Climate	more	less	less
Cold Climate	less	more	more

If an animal is born with a fairly good constitution and is getting wholesome food, fresh air, clean fresh water, sunshine, and moderate exercise, it should enjoy a healthy and long life. However, in today's highly chemicalized society, pollution from farm and industry make this goal harder and harder to accomplish.

Basic Dog Diet

The average diet for an adult dog should be by volume approximately fifty percent cooked whole grains, twenty-five percent animal food in the form of beef, rabbit, lamb, or chicken, and twenty-five percent steamed fresh vegetables in season and grown locally.

Of course, the diet will differ with the type of dog and with each individual. We should be careful about making generalities. It's like the fellow who drowned walking across a stream that averaged two feet deep. Generally speaking, the smaller breeds are more yang. Chihuahuas, for example, because of their background, have an affinity for fowl. They like chicken better than do most breeds of dogs. Again, I would try to stay fairly close to the standard macrobiotic diet. As I mentioned earlier, I also take into consideration where this animal came from originally and what it originally did.

It's hard to generalize. We have to use our intuition to a large extent. Take the dachshund. He was originally used as a burrowing dog, hunting for animals that burrow. He's a very tough little guy. Once a lady here in Texas with a St. Bernard called me during a very hot spell. She said, "I want you to tell me what to do for this dog. I must know." I said, "The first thing you have got to do is go get some plywood and build a great big box and then ship him back to Switzerland where he belongs." Taking a dog that was built for cold weather with this great big coat on him and putting him down here in this Texas heat and feeding him a high-protein diet just burns him up.

A less drastic solution would be to add something cooling to the diet, like tofu and raw vegetables such as cabbage. That helps to cool them down. I would also cut down on protein. Protein is very warming and makes animals hot.

Working dogs were selected for their capacity for tremendous amounts of exercise. If we change their environment, we should not keep them on a high-protein diet. That is like putting high octane gasoline in a car that's not made for it. We need to calm them down. For example, if an animal didn't have the opportunity to run every day like he would in a natural environment, I would use something like tofu for the protein part of the diet to calm him down. If you give him large amounts of animal protein and then put him in a confined environment, you are asking for an explosion.

A lower protein diet—good-quality protein such as that in grain, beans, and bean products—will solve many problems. If your pet is hyperactive, I would definitely change from animal to vegetable protein, with the exception of white-meat fish.

If you are training the animal for a working season and are going to have him outdoors, you can begin to increase his exercise and increase the amount of protein in his diet. Actually, the amount of high-energy food determines the amount of exercise he'll want. You could then use up to 25 percent red meat instead of vegetable protein.

Again, I keep referring to the animal's original constitution and the conditions under which it lives. The questions we must ask ourselves are, What's the environment like? What was the animal bred for? What's its background? What was its original food? What was its purpose originally?

The collie, for example, was bred as a sheepherding dog and was traditionally fed oats and whey. It was primarily vegetarian—a very docile animal that took things easy. That was a more yin diet, suited to its more yin lifestyle. If today you take a collie and feed him a more yang diet—high in animal protein—and then confine him in a small place—which also has a tight, compact yang quality—you are asking for trouble. In addition to bad teeth and skin problems, many times bad eyesight will develop. The liver is the major detoxifying organ of the body, and it tries to throw off nutritional excess. But if it can't handle all this toxic material, we begin to see a discharge, especially in the eye, maybe just in the corners. This is an overflow. In Oriental medicine, eye trouble is associated with trouble in the liver.

If we look at the animal from the front to the rear, the intake system is the mouth, and the exhaust system is the rectum. The next thing after eye trouble that we will see is problems in the exhaust system. We may see thinning of the coat or skin problems near the base of the tail or in that general area. If we recognize that this is probably diet-caused, then we can modify the diet and help reverse the condition. The processed fat that the body is not prepared to handle is a big factor here. If the animal is in a situation where we can't get that done, then I try to add something to burn some of that stuff off. But I try to purify the diet as much as possible. It's not in the best interest of the animal to have a shot of cortisone or some penicillin to treat the symptoms. It just makes things worse.

Basic Cat Diet

The maintenance diet for the average healthy cat should be by volume about twenty-five percent cooked grain, fifty percent animal food in the form of beef, organ meat, and/or fish, and twenty-five percent steamed, fresh vegetables. That's a lot higher more protein than we'd recommend for a person or a dog. But then they are more compact or, as we would say in Oriental philosophy, more yang. Therefore their energy requirements are higher.

When we consider the cat, the first thing to remember is that it is a domestic animal that has lived with man for at least twenty thousand years. They have adapted pretty well to people as they have evolved. The cat is more independent than the dog. They are more attached to places than to people. They can become attached to people, but their attitude is more like, "I'll let you love me," rather than "I have to have your love."

I never cease to be amazed at cats. I watch them and my own cats because I enjoy observing their idiosyncrasies and the things they do to manipulate me. They are quite good at getting what they want. They can fake all kinds of things to get you to do what they want you to do.

A good, clean diet should contain good, clean ingredients. As I've said, this would include whole grains, meat or fish, and vegetables. You can use a little poultry, but poultry is not the ideal food for cats, because they would not eat very much chicken in the wild every day. They would eat a bird every once in a while. We have to look at their diet from that standpoint. The vegetables they would have gotten would have been in the stomachs of the mice or other small rodents they captured and ate. From looking at their teeth patterns, we see that cats need about fifty to sixty percent concentrated protein. That would be primarily meat or fish.

One of the great foods for cats is rabbit. I never cease to be amazed at how well rabbit fits into the picture. We tried feeding rabbit to cats in some eating experiments and were able to watch their bodies respond. It was fascinating to see how cats reacted when they ate the way they probably would in a natural environment. Not only did their bodies change, but their attitudes changed also.

In a modern household, where the cat is not hunting for itself, I like to give it about twenty-five percent fresh vegetables, usually steamed, but also boiled, or cooked from time to time in other ways. Then to balance the diet, especially to ensure a steady source of trace minerals, I would add a little seaweed every day, because seaweed is an important source of trace minerals. This diet is the end result of much observation and many feeding experiments. Over the years I've found that cats really thrive on this approach.

For protein, beef is generally available and appropriate. I will use chicken, since we live in a chicken culture today. But I don't like chicken as much, because it has a tendency to produce more mucus than beef and it's not so easily digested. We found a world of difference in our feeding experiments between giving the cat chicken and rabbit. The cats fed on rabbit took less food. My older cat, Luther, would fake me out in order to get rabbit. He would make out like he was starved to death if he didn't get any rabbit. I would put other food down for him to eat. He would walk over and wait and wait as if to say, "I don't understand why you are putting that stuff over here. This is where the rabbit goes." He would almost talk to me and try to tell me he just had to have that rabbit. I was giving him chicken and other things, even beef, but he was trying to tell me that they were not good enough. Then we worked out a deal where he had rabbit on certain days. It was amazing that he knew on which days we were going to give him rabbit.

Although I had a large number of cats to work with, as with people, if you know them well, you can tell what they are enthusiastic about. Certain individuals like certain things. I used to have some Siamese kittens that were litter mates. One of the kittens would eat whatever I put out very well. It enjoyed a tremendous variety and never fussed. The other one would squall as if it were being hit. It was angry with me if I didn't feed it what it wanted.

I made many interesting observations. I noticed that if I ate my lunch in the vicinity of the cats, they would come around and beg to have some of my food. They liked watching me eat. Fulton will eat most anything he sees me eating, and he likes to talk me into giving him something from my plate. He will not always relish it, but he will at least taste it and give me a look as if to say, "No, I don't want any of that."

I am simply amazed at the things he will try. He likes different melons, especially watermelon, and he will eat cantaloupe.

Giving your cat variety helps develop a close relationship with the animal. And giving the cat some of your own food creates a bond of love just as it does between people. If you are eating something and they are acting like they want some, spit a little bit of it into their bowl and mix it with the other food. They seem to love it, even plain brown rice. I have found that pre-chewing increased their ability to digest.

There may be some little parts of vegetables on your plate that you won't eat, such as the roots of onions or the tips of scallions. You can take those and wash them real good, chop them up fine, and mix them in with the cat's food, and this gives them variety. In nature, they would get this sort of food from the stomachs of small rodents.

For grains, I like to use brown rice especially, as well as oats and barley. Barley soup, mixed with other grains, seems to be a very wonderful thing for cats. The barley makes them feel better. I have found that just a little barley soup added to their other food breaks the monotony of the feeding regime.

In my feeding trials, I noticed that you have to be careful that the animal is digesting the grain properly. If the brown rice is not carefully cooked, it will come through undigested. You can tell when this is happening by examining the stool. If there are grains in the stool, it shows that there is incomplete absorption. If you see that grain come through in the stool, you may want to grind the grain before you cook it, or blend it after you cook it so it's in smaller particles. The cat's digestive system is short, like that of the dog, and grain goes through pretty hurriedly.

I like to feed my cats cornmeal, especially that which is freshly ground. I make what people would call cornbread for the animals and mix this in with the food, and they really love it.

The vegetables should be steamed and blended or chopped into small particles. I go with the seasons as much as possible. I give my cats root vegetables in the wintertime such as carrots, rutabagas, and turnips. As the summertime comes along, I go more with the leafy green vegetables such as cab-bage, collards, and lettuce. They particularly go for cabbage, if it is chopped very fine. I find that it acts like a broom to clean out their systems. I feed it raw or lightly steamed.

Squash is also wonderful. I told a lady once to put squash in the diet of her cat, and she was insulted. She said her cat would never eat that. I said to just try adding a tiny bit and see if we could introduce it gradually. She now calls that cat a squashaholic. She says when she is cooking squash, he will jump up by the stove and knock the pan off with his paw to get it before it's done. He loves squash.

Fruits, too, can be given to the cat in small amounts, es-pecially in the summertime. Not all cats like fruit, but some do.

For seaweed, I use a pinch of powdered kelp. It contains about six times as much calcium as cow's milk and it's in an organic form that is more digestible than dairy food. I have also found that cats love nori, the thin, wafer-like black or dark green seaweed that is commonly used in making sushi spirals. It has a fishy flavor that seems to attract them.

Occasionally, I will let the cat fast. I'll skip feeding him once every two weeks. I don't like to fast cats as a regular thing. It's a good idea to fast a dog once a week, but cats seem to require more regularity. As opposed to fasting, I will feed them lightly once every ten days to two weeks just a quarter of a meal. Reducing the amount of food like this every few weeks gives the cat's G.I. tract a rest. The next meal or next day, the cat is really anxious to get her food.

In general, cats will eat less than dogs. They are not as prone to overeating. There are dogs that will eat until they make themselves sick. I have never seen that in a cat.

A small kitten, about eight weeks old, should be fed a minimum of three times a day. I would feed it more if I could, But a lot of people are working and can't do that. If you are in a situation like that, it makes sense to leave some food out when you are gone, because the kitten will get hungry during the day. Eventually you can cut back on the number of times you feed it. I find generally that cats need to be fed more of-ten than dogs. I only feed a dog once a day. But a cat thrives better on at least one small meal and one large meal daily. A cat can get along pretty well if it's fed once a day if you provide little tidbits at other times of the day. Giving tidbits like this is fine.

For fish, I like to use white-meat fish rather than red-meat or blue-skin fish. It is less oily and fatty and also less polluted. Tuna picks up mercury. As opposed to freshwater fish that may be in contaminated water, deep ocean fish that swim near the bottom of the sea are cleaner.

The Vegetarian Cat

Sometimes people ask me if a cat can be a complete vegetarian. Cats eating a vegetarian diet do very well. I have several of them that belong to people who are vegetarian and don't want to feed them meat, poultry, or fish. Cats like this will also eat bean sprouts and nuts. Alfalfa sprouts, chopped really fine, are a favorite of theirs.

When I experimented with a total vegetarian diet for cats, I found that their requirements for protein seemed to lessen. I like to use tofu and chickpeas. I haven't been able to determine why it is, but chickpeas seem to be the bean of choice, even more than aduki beans, which cats also like. They should be well cooked and then blended so they can be mixed in with the rest of the cat's food. Tofu and seitan—or wheat gluten—can also be used as protein sources.

It was interesting to me to observe vegetarian cats. I said to myself, "This animal in nature would catch a mouse." I noticed that cats like this were often getting protein from another source. They would be very keen to small insects, and catch and eat any they found. I think they were trying to tell me something.

I have people come in who are total vegetarians. I have people come who don't eat meat but who eat fish. Others eat only fruits and juices. I try to work with all of them and respect their ways of life. I do find, as a rule, that animals that are strictly vegetarian are a little more laid back. I would generally expect this to be the case. They are more on the yin side. They are more relaxed, less aggressive.

There are animals that have personality problems. This is something being studied now. We are finding that different animals fit different personality patterns. For example, there is the pulsatilla cat; that's a cat that can't let go. It can't let the owner get away from them. It clings as if to say, "Something bad is going to happen to me. I just can't stand to let somebody else touch me." We can give that cat a little pulsatilla and it begins to relax. As I will explain in the next book in this series, we are using homeopathic remedies. We find they work. Both cats and birds respond beautifully to homeopathic remedies.

Diet and the Emotions

A common sign of dietary imbalance or environmental stress is irritability. Irritability has a lot to do with the attitude of the animal. I find that an animal with a skin problem and digestive problems has a tendency to have a more unhappy attitude, if not an aggressive one. If there are two or three other animals in the family, sometimes the dog—or often the cat—resents the other animals and has a bad attitude. If you can work that out through diet, the animal begins to improve. Her whole attitude changes. She becomes more peaceful.

Last week I had a very belligerent little schnauzer. When we solved its skin problem, its whole attitude changed. It had eaten a poor diet for a couple of years. But in a very short time this animal changed. I just cooled him down by adding tofu and fresh leafy green vegetables to his diet, and then I resolved the skin problem with a homeopathic remedy. The woman was most happy with that because she has never seen her Schnauzer so loving. This happened because the animal felt better. She didn't feel irritated all the time. She is an absolutely beautiful animal now and is doing very well.

Like many people, this woman was working and found it difficult to prepare fresh food for her pet. It's hard to convince someone like this to change all at once, so I told her to add some fresh vegetables to her dog's usual canned food. I also told her to add just a small amount of meat, only a tea-spoonful of very lean raw beef. This acted like a catalyst, ena-bling the little dog's body to burn off some of the toxins that it had been accumulating.

Over time, you will learn to monitor your dog or cat's condition and change its diet to address imbalances effective-ly. Your animal will reward you with its beauty and sweet disposition.

10
Grooming, Exercising, Bathing, Immunizing, Neutering, and Spaying

The thing I remember most from the early training my Grandmother gave me was how she taught me to care about the comfort of all the animals on the farm. She had come from the North, and I suppose her early childhood experience of surviving cold winters on the prairies of Nebraska in a dugout (a home dug in the ground) influenced her, for she was a great believer in barns. On cold nights, she would not be satisfied until all animals on the place were bedded down. She would be sure the chickens were closed up and out of the weather.

Our dogs and cats were well taken care of, because they had shelter and natural foods. They shared our way of life. This is the way that life—human and animal—has evolved for generations, as far as I can see; animals have shared human fate in both good and bad times. The present is no exception. Humans, with our his scientific advancement, have become separated from the earth, our mother. We have done this by turning away from nature, chemicalizing the soil and filling our bodies with drugs and preservatives and processed foods. By doing this, we are severing our bonds with the earth. As a result we are seeing a decline in the natural immune system in both ourselves and our animals. The animals under our care and protection seem to be our weathervanes. By observing them, we can see where we are headed. It is not an encouraging picture. We use vaccines to stimulate the body to produce resistance to disease, but what if the immune system is incapable of responding to the stimulus? It is my belief that this is what we are seeing today in both animals and man.

What can we do? As so many people have discovered, we must return to a more natural way of life. This is especially true in the areas of food and environment, both prenatal and postnatal. Our modern approach to health has largely overlooked the prenatal life where the constitution is formed. The natural resistance is set up in this formative phase of life, continues to shape and influence the entire life span. Unless we make drastic changes, we are set on a course of self-destruction.

Grooming the Cat

Cats are rather fastidious animals and do a good job of cleaning themselves. They can clean their whole bodies, including the fur, except inside their ears and at the point of the chin. It is a good idea to clean inside the cat's ears with olive oil on a cotton-covered applicator stick or a Q-Tip. Thinner oils dissolve thicker oils, so the olive oil will help remove any excess wax that has built up. This should be done at least twice a week. Daily is better. If it is done daily, there will usually be very little to do. Just moisten the cotton with olive oil and clean the inside of the ear. Any accumulation of black material in the ear should be viewed with caution. This would call for more oil in the ear and a more thorough cleaning. If the black material persists, the cat has ear mites, and you should consider adding some type of ear preparation that contains an insecticide to your ear-cleaning routine for a few days, though I recommend that you use a more natural product. One that contains five percent pyrethin, a natural insecticide, would be good for cleaning out any ear mites present. If the black material persists despite your efforts, it would be a good idea to seek professional help.

Baby kittens are cleaned by the mother's licking and grooming. She does this with her tongue, which serves as a small brush. When she licks the anus and the penis or vulva, it stimulates the baby to urinate or defecate. The mother cat eats these wastes for sanitary reasons, and this helps to keep her babies bright and healthy. If for some reason your mother cat can't do this or if the kitten is an orphan, you should take care of this chore yourself. You can do this by moistening a piece of cotton with warm water and then stroking the anus and penis or vulva, and the baby will more than likely discharge at that time.

If you start early, when the cat is a small kitten, your cat will, in all probability, accept your help with the grooming without protest and even enjoy it. If your cat is a long-haired variety, I suggest you get a slicker brush. This is a small brush with metal teeth that are bent just right for grooming longer coats. On the other hand, if your animal has a short-haired coat, a softer brush or a grooming glove would be best. If you spend a few minutes each day grooming your cat, you will be aware if something begins to go wrong. This is a good time for massaging the animal, too. If your animal suddenly develops a lot of fleas, it would be good to check around the anus for tapeworm segments. These will look like small grains of white rice on the area around the anus or sometimes on the bedding when the animal sleeps. This is not so likely to happen if you are including some ground pumpkin seed in the diet and possibly some Kyolic garlic (a deodorized garlic supplement) at least twice a week.

If tapeworms develop, it is very hard to get rid of them with worming alone. You almost have to control fleas to control tapeworms, as the tapeworm goes through the flea as an intermediate host.

Brushing the cat can be beneficial to both the cat and to you. This is especially true if there is mutual love and affection. Electromagnetic energy passes from the meridians along the back of the cat, through the fingertips of the person doing the brushing, and back to the cat. You can see this energy as sparks by brushing a cat in a very dark room. There is a healthy exchange of energy in both directions if both animal and human are healthy. The energy tends to flow both ways. Therefore, if you are ill, it's better for you not to brush the animal. On the other hand, you can receive some good energy from a healthy cat if your own vitality is low.

The scientific community is reporting on the possible transfer of some exotic diseases between cats and people. I would think there would be more likelihood of this if the cat were allowed to roam the neighborhood, where it could come in contact with toxins or infectious agents. This could occur by mechanical means, too. By keeping your animal clean and restricting such contacts, you can reduce this danger to a minimum.

Bathing the Cat

Bathing an uncooperative or unwilling cat can be an ordeal. Common sense is called for. We would not think of not keeping ourselves clean. Therefore, if we are to share our quarters and possibly our bed with an animal, it should be understood that the animal must be kept clean, too. Sanitation is the very first line of defense in disease prevention after proper diet.

There is one word of caution about bathing. Too much bathing is worse than no bathing at all. Too much bathing seems to wash out minerals, vitamins, and some of the protection the animal has against disease. I suggest one bath for a household pet every seven to ten days. See section below on flea collars.

Bathing the Dog

On the farm, we never bathed our dogs at all. The only baths they got was in the creek or pond, which they did on their own, especially in summertime. But certainly, if you have dogs in the house with you, they will need to be washed from time to time. But if we overbathe them, they lose some protective oils from the skin. Puppies should not be bathed until they have acquired some immunity, because they seem to have a natural protection in the coat. If you wash that out, you make them more susceptible to diseases. The mother initially cleans and licks them; that's the natural way. I like for them to have the second series of shots before they're bathed.

For general bathing, I recommend a natural soap. Be careful of flea products that contain strong insecticides. Each one causes us to use a little stronger one, and after a while we have a monstrous flea. I heard a man say on the radio, "Maybe the only way to kill 'em is to hit 'em with a hammer." That's true. I like to bathe dogs with a natural soap once every ten days to two weeks. That should be sufficient for an animal that spends most of the time in the house.

If the dog has a really strong odor, it's a good idea to check the anal glands that lie on either side of the anus. Many times that gland is not properly discharging, causing the odor. If that is the problem, then I look first at the diet. If the dog is eating a lot of smelly food, you get a lot of smell in the skin. I like to put vegetables in the diet. That will do more for cleaning up the skin and making a dog smell fresh than anything. I will use raw or lightly steamed vegetables such as cabbage, swiss chard, kale, and other leafy vegetables in season.

Vegetables have a cleansing effect on the skin. On every side of every hair follicle is a sebaceous gland. This secretes sebum. That's primarily the way it's done. If those glands are open and secreting, they secrete nice oil that makes the coat shiny. If those glands are not functioning properly, there's a stoppage, and we get heavier oils from there and that gland secretes that. Then the skin begins itching. The next thing you know, your pet has a skin problem. The way to avoid that is through modifying the diet. You get good shiny coats on animals from oils in grains. Sometimes it takes several months for the animal to eliminate the old fats in its system.

Flea Collars

I discourage the use of flea collars and insecticides. By and large they don't work. I have seen third-degree burns on animals caused by flea collars. This seems to occur in warm, damp weather. I can't imagine a more cruel thing than having to wear something fixed around the neck that is constantly burning. Flea collars and insecticides particularly affect the liver. The liver is the organ chiefly responsible for activating the immune system. Is it any wonder that we are seeing the lack of immune response in both animals and humans, with all the chemicals we use?

I have seen an electronic flea collar that works by emitting a sound that fleas and ticks can't tolerate. My very first question on that device is, What is it doing to the sensitive ears of the cat or dog wearing it? It will be a while before we know the answers.

Dipping cats should be viewed with caution. If you feel you must dip, use only natural products.

Grooming the Dog

The many breeds of dogs, with their almost endless variety of hair coats and qualities makes it difficult to make a general rule for grooming and cleaning. Common sense is the best approach. The mother dog starts to groom the puppies by licking and cleaning much the same way as the mother cat. She will continue this licking and grooming right up to weaning time. Her licking and grooming the body orifices of the puppies stimulates them to urinate and defecate. Like the mother cat, she also eats the puppies' waste. Usually the mother dog will do some grooming up until she stops nursing the puppies. Some will continue beyond. I once knew a dog that seemed to think it was her duty to clean and pick fleas off her offspring even after they had grown up.

Some of the factors to consider in grooming are: Is this to be an outside or an inside dog? Is it short- or long-haired? What is the original purpose of the breed? Are we going to want to change the animal's purpose (for example, to change a retriever into a house dog)?

Immunizations

We have to continue to depend on vaccines to some extent. At our clinic, we start out by giving puppies a combined vaccine for distemper, hepatitis, and leptospirosis. Leptospirosis prevents a disease known fifty years ago as Stuttgart disease (because it was discovered in Stuttgart, Germany), but it's no longer a threat to us. I've only seen one case in the last ten years. However, evidence is now surfacing that these combined vaccines are not in the best interest of the animal. We should give the immune system a chance to respond to one stimulus before we introduce it to another. I like to spread out the vaccinations myself—to give them separately. Then we have parvo virus, a virus that was at one time known as panleukopenia in cats. It's still a cat disease, but in about 1979, this virus seemed to modify itself and began to attack dogs, and we had quite a death loss in the United States.

We are watching it, because we had one heck of a time when parvo came in. It seems now to have subsided but at first it hit dogs of every kind and size. The death loss was almost unbelievable. The epidemic almost overwhelmed us.

There is also corona virus; it's a virus that produces a Parvo like syndrome. They have produced a vaccine for it now. We are viewing it with caution, using it where we feel it's necessary, where there may be a threat to the animal.

By the same token, I'm wondering if we haven't created a monstrous condition by the widespread use of antibiotics. "Anti" means against, and "biotics" means life. And through the widespread use of antibiotics, it seems to me we've created super-viruses. There was a radio appeal just this week by a Dr. Metcalf at the University of Illinois against the use of strong pesticides. He said we are creating a super bug because we continue to use these strong pesticides.

By the same token, with the widespread use of antibiotics in our food, I feel that we have created very unwholesome conditions. Still, we have to depend somewhat on vaccines; it's better to stimulate the immune system to some degree because we've seen good evidence that if we didn't have some kind of immunity, we would just wipe our animals out in a hurry. Eventually, if we could strengthen the immune system through the use of good food that is not contaminated with pesticides and chemicals, that would be the best. In the meantime, we have to live where we are. We now also have available to us the nosodes for several of these diseases.

We should be aware that there is such a thing as a bad reaction from these vaccines. Some veterinarians are working to minimize these reactions. One of the things that we like to use to offset these reactions is a homeopathic remedy called iachesis. Dr. Pitcairn reported this in some of his work. It helps the body discharge any untoward effects, reducing the chance of having a bad reaction to the vaccine. Again, I like to stagger those vaccines, to give one every two weeks or so to give the animal time to adjust and for us to identify any severe reactions. Then I can work with the animal, as opposed to giving them all at once and wondering what's going to happen. If all the vaccines are given at once, the animal might also develop depression or skin problems.

One of the principles in homeopathy is that the body needs time to react. The homeopathic remedies work a lot like a vaccine. A vaccine is like a small dose of the disease. Take apis mel, for example. Apis means bee sting. This remedy is very good for swelling. Homeopathy is based on the Law of Similars and was introduced by Dr. Hahnemann, the founder of modern homeopathy. Of course, it goes back into Ayurvedic medicine, which is traditional Indian medicine. What it means is that you take something that would create a similar condition, a minute amount of it, and give it to the animal. This stimulates the body to respond of its own accord. For example, we would use apis in a 6X potency. That means you would dilute one drop of the bee sting material in nine drops of water, and you would repeat that process six times. Actually you would be getting very, very little of the bee sting material.

The most important resistance to disease in the animal comes from natural immunity. This immunity is acquired from the colostrum, the first mother's milk. We wait a week or ten days after weaning before we begin the vaccines.

I ran an animal shelter once for eighteen months, and during this time I took six puppies and gave three of them vaccines and three of them distilled water. Then I observed them. In that shelter, it was almost impossible to keep them from being exposed to distemper. During the follow-up, I discovered that the vaccinated puppies lived, and the majority of the unvaccinated puppies died. This was good evidence, as far as I was concerned, that the vaccines were working. I instituted a program at that time that is still used by the SPCA and the city pound here in Dallas of immunizing animals I felt were adoptable as soon as they came in the door, rather than waiting and sending them out with no vaccine at all. I had to deal with the problem myself, and it was heartrending to have people adopt a puppy that seemed all nice and healthy and then have them see it die of distemper. That's why I began the program.

Spaying and Neutering

I am in full agreement with Dr. Michael Fox when he says that a neutered animal is a happier pet. The best time to spay a cat is after she has had her first heat period. That indicates that she is sexually mature. Though this is the ideal time, it does not mean that older cats cannot be successfully spayed. They can very well.

The best time to neuter a male cat is when he is sexually mature. This is usually at about six months of age. He will usually begin to spray at about this time, and that means he is beginning to mark his territory.

Cats live under the kingdom law. That means that the mature male cat begins to consider the home his territory for sexual purposes, and he marks it by spraying with urine. Any female within that marked territory he considers his. It may be your neighbor's beautiful purebred show animal, but to him she is his female. If a tom cat is free to roam, he will fight to defend his territory. If any female within his territory wanders to the outer edge, he whips her and runs her back. Any male cat that comes into his territory will be fought. Even small or baby kittens are considered a threat and may be killed and eaten.

Dogs, on the other hand, evolved from the law of the pack. Dogs tend to return to this law if allowed to roam free. They tend to join a pack and hunt and scavenge together. If a fight develops and one dog is down and crying out, they all tend to join in and destroy the one that is down.

Neutered dogs rarely join a pack. There are exceptions to this, but they are not common. This is because the sexual drive stimulus has been removed, and they have become more peaceful (more yin). Spayed females would have even less tendency to join the pack, because they are already more yin (more peaceful) naturally than the male.

The food requirements for a spayed female or a neutered male change after the surgery. This is because the body demands less yang energy (aggressive energy) directed toward the sexual drive. However, there is an adjustment time for the animal's body following surgery.

If we are aware of this adjustment period and are careful with the feeding during this crucial time, we can lessen or eliminate the tendency toward obesity. On the other hand, if we continue to feed the animal high-energy foods with preservatives and insecticides we can look for some type of problem to develop. This is especially true if the food is left out all the time.

It is especially important to realize that the newly spayed or neutered animal's requirements for body maintenance will be different now. There are two things to keep in mind. First, the animal will not be aware of the lessened body requirements because of residual sex hormones in the body. Second, because of this, the animal may have a tendency to get fat.

We can help the animal through this difficult period by controlling the food intake. It is better to keep the animal just a little hungry than to overfeed it. And this is a good time to add some herbs to the diet. A small amount of red raspberry leaves and squaw vine for the female, or sarsaparilla and a homeopathic ginseng, could be used.

Listening to Your Pet

In the sequel to this book, I will discuss the specific measures and remedies I use for specific conditions, using dietary adjustments, herbs, homeopathy, and other natural treatments. In this first book, I have simply tried to share with you my love of animals and the natural world, as well as a little of what I know about raising healthy pets. With the accelerated pace of life today, I'm afraid that we are losing touch with nature and this knowledge, exemplified by my grandmother, is rapidly vanishing. As I have stated repeatedly in this book, animals are our weathervanes, pointing us toward either the sunshine about to break out or the stormclouds gathering overhead. Animals have a wealth of love to share, as well as an intuitive sense of approaching danger. By listening to your dog or cat, you can learn to enhance your own health and well-being.

Resources

Dr. Norman Ralston is director of the LBJ Animal Clinic in Dallas. For information, including consultations by phone, please contact:

LBJ Animal Clinic
12500 Lake June
Balch Springs, TX 75180
(214) 391-7186

One Peaceful World is an international information network and friendship society devoted to the realization of one healthy, peaceful world. Activities include educational and spiritual tours, assemblies and forums, international food aid and development, and publishing. Membership is $30/year for individuals and $50 for families and includes a subscription to the One Peaceful World Newsletter and a free book from One Peaceful World Press. For further information, contact:

One Peaceful World
Box 10
Becket, MA 01223
(413) 623–2322
Fax (413) 623–8827

Recommended Reading

1. Esko, Edward. *Notes from the Boundless Frontier* (One Peaceful World Press, 1992).

2. Esko, Edward. *The Pulse of Life* (One Peaceful World Press, 1994).

3. Esko, Wendy. *Rice Is Nice* (One Peaceful World Press, 1995).

4. Esko, Wendy. *Soup du Jour* (One Peaceful World Press, 1996).

5. Jack, Gale and Alex Jack, *Amber Waves of Grain* (Japan Publications, 1993).

6. Jack, Gale, *Promenade Home: Macrobiotics and Women's Health* (Japan Publications, 1988).

7. Kushi, Michio. *Basic Shiatsu* (with Edward Esko, One Peaceful World Press, 1995).

8. Kushi, Michio. *Forgotten Worlds* (with Edward Esko, One Peaceful World Press, 1992).

9. Kushi, Michio. *One Peaceful World* (with Alex Jack, St. Martin's Press, 1987).

10. Kushi, Michio. *Spiritual Journey* (with Edward Esko, One Peaceful World Press, 1995).

For a free catalog of books on natural health, diet, and the environment, please write One Peaceful World Press, P. O. Box 10, Becket, MA 01223.

About the Authors

Norman Ralston, D.V.M., is director of the LBJ Animal Clinic in Dallas, Texas. He has served as president of the American Holistic Veterinary Association, the Dallas S.P.C.A., and other professional and civic organizations. His unique approach to pet care has been featured in the *Dallas Morning News, PM Magazine, East West Journal,* and other publications and on radio and television. He lives with his wife in the Dallas area.

Gale Jack is a macrobiotic cooking teacher, author of *Promenade Home* and *Amber Waves of Grain,* and a former resident of Dallas. She lives with her family in Becket, Massachusetts.